Natural Remedies: A Manual

Phylis Austin
Agatha M. Thrash, M.D.
Calvin L. Thrash, Jr., M.D.

FAMILY HEALTH PUBLICATIONS
13062 MUSGROVE HWY.
SUNFIELD, MICH. 48890

Library of Congress Cataloging in Publication Data

Austin, Phylis,
  Natural remedies.

  Bibliography: p.
  Includes index.
  1. Naturopathy—Handbooks, manuals, etc.
2. Therapeutics, Physiological—Handbooks, manuals, etc.
I. Thrash, Agatha M., 1931- . II. Thrash, Calvin L., 1928- . III. Yuchi Pines
Institute. IV. Title.
RZ440.A9   1983   615.5'35   82-24703
ISBN: 0-942658-05-1

TABLE OF CONTENTS

Acne Vulgaris 1
Acrodermatitis Enteropathica 2
Angina Pectoris 3
Aphthous Ulcers 5
Arthritis 6
Asthma 10
Athlete's Foot 17
Backache 19
Bad Breath 22
Bedwetting 24
Bell's Palsy 26
Bronchiectasis 28
Bronchitis 29
Buerger's Disease 31
Bursitis 33
Celiac Disease 34
Chiggers 36
Colic 37
Cradle Cap 40
Crohn's Disease 41
Cystitis 43
Diverticulitis and Diverticulosis 46
Dysmenorrhea 47
Gallstones 51
Gas 54
Gout 58
Hay Fever 62
Hiccups 63
Impetigo Contagiosa 65
Influenza 66
Intermittent Claudication 68
Irritable Bowel Syndrome 70
Kidney Stones 73
Mastitis 76
Meniere's Disease 78
Migraine 80
Muscle Cramps 84
Osteoporosis 87

Parkinson's Disease 92
Peptic Ulcer 97
Poison Ivy 101
Pruritus Ani 103
Raynaud's Phenomenon 105
Restless Leg Syndrome 109
Rheumatoid Arthritis 110
Sinusitis 115
Tennis Elbow 118
Thrombophlebitis—See Venous Thrombosis
Thrush 119
Ulcerative Colitis 120
Vaginitis 124
Varicose Veins 126
Venous Thrombosis 130
Warts 132
Appendix A 135
Appendix B 138
Appendix C 139
Appendix D 140
Appendix E 141
Appendix F 142
Bibliography 143
Index 161

ACNE VULGARIS

Acne vulgaris is probably the most common skin disorder in the United States. The face, chest, shoulders and back are the primary sites of involvement. Although acne vulgaris is usually benign and limited to the adolescent years, the cystic form can be chronic, widespread, and disfiguring. Some recent studies cast doubt on food connections in acne, such as chocolate, fats and sweets. Most experienced dermatologists and acne sufferers will attest to the value of avoidance of these items, however. In a population nearly 100% of whom are consuming large quantities of these nutrients, one would not expect relatively minor variations in the offending agents to make much difference statistically. But in a population such as the Eskimos, who had eaten little or no sweets prior to 1950 and then had a veritable explosion of sugar intake (from 26 pounds per person per year to 104 pounds in 8 years), acne is now occurring in epidemic proportions. (532)

TREATMENT

1. Stress may play a role in worsening acne. (483) Neutralize stress with daily out-of-doors exercise.

2. Cleansing the skin every four to six hours will discourage bacterial growth. Washing may be done with or without a washcloth. Using lukewarm water, lather gently and thoroughly for one minute. Rinse in lukewarm water. Repeat a second time.

3. Many cosmetics and lotions contain chemicals that may aggravate acne. Nia K. Terezakis, M.D. states that some of the most popular commercial skin care products may be the greatest culprits in skin problems. Dr. Terezakis suggests compresses of cornstarch, baking soda or a combination of the two. (484)

4. In the same article, Dr. Terezakis suggests the use of 100% cotton clothing and bed linen rather than synthetic fabrics.

5. Do not squeeze pimples or blackheads as this often pushes the blackhead down into the skin. (485)

6. Shampoo nightly or twice a week. Keep hair off the face either by short haircuts or pinning up.

7. Do not prop your hands against your face or even touch the face with the fingers; always use a clean tissue, even to scratch an itch.

8. Sunshine will help acne by increasing the peeling of the surface keratin and preventing blockage of the skin glands. Sufficient

sun to induce a slight reddening of the skin is recommended. The relaxation associated with sun bathing may also benefit acne. (486)

9. Food sensitivities are known to cause acne. (473) Milk, (487) chocolate, nuts, peanut, and egg are common offenders. (473)

10. Salt restriction may be quite beneficial. (488) Avoid high sodium foods such as potato chips, catsup, french fries, and dairy products for a two week trial period.

11. A fat-free diet (See Appendix C) has been found to be helpful. (488)

12. Goldenseal tea compresses may be applied to inflamed lesions.

13. Drink sufficient water to keep the urine pale to assist in keeping the secretions thinner and more readily discharged.

14. Some people will get pimples and a rash from their own saliva which may drool at night onto their pillow.

15. Avoid tight collars and helmets.

ACRODERMATITIS ENTEROPATHICA

Acrodermatitis enteropathica is characterized by dermatitis, diarrhea, and loss of hair. Two-thirds of patients have a family history of the disease and genetically susceptible infants who are not breast-fed generally develop symptoms in the first four to ten weeks of life. Breast-feeding is protective; onset of acrodermatitis enteropathica is generally within a week or so of the introduction of cow's milk into the diet. (499)

TREATMENT

1. Breast feed infants.

2. Aspirin, calcium, and soy milk protein impair zinc absorption and should be avoided. (498)

3. Zinc supplements dramatically reverse symptoms. Daily doses of 50 mg. of zinc for infants, 150 mg. for children, (500) and as much as 220 mg. for adults have been given. Upon administration of zinc, behavioral changes are the first sign of improvement to be noticed. Infants become less irritable, less dependent, and better sleepers within one to two days after zinc therapy is begun. Normal appetite returns about the same time and skin clearing

often begins in two to three days, but several weeks may be required for complete clearing. Diarrhea ceases in a few days. Hair growth is noticeable in two to three weeks and body growth in six to eight weeks. (499)

4. Use a diet high in zinc, using such foods as legumes and whole grain products. One adult female took a dandelion brew for two years during which time she had improvement in her symptoms, felt to be due to the dietary supplementation of zinc provided by the dandelions. (501)

5. Zinc-deficient animals show increased susceptibility to bacterial and yeast infection and these should be guarded against. Keep the immune system functioning at its peak by regular rest and exercise, a simple diet, and regularity.

ANGINA PECTORIS

Angina pectoris is a sensation of discomfort in the chest and adjoining areas caused by an inadequate supply of oxygen to the heart muscle. The typical patient is male, in his fifties or early sixties. Approximately 80% are men. (2) About 90% of cases of angina are due to coronary atherosclerosis (thickening of the walls of the blood vessels, with narrowing of the opening through which the blood flows). Often at least one of the three major coronary arteries are closed down 80% before angina develops, but in most cases more than one of the three major arteries are involved. (1)

Patients do not describe their discomfort as pain, but rather as a pressure, constriction, smothering, heaviness, choking or squeezing sensation, or even indigestion. (20)

The pain of angina is generally located in the mid- or upper third of the sternum, but it is frequently noted in the lower sternum, one or both sides of the chest (most commonly the left), the arms (generally the left), and into the neck and jaw, or even the teeth. (3) The pain may be mild or severe, and is often controlled by slowing down or stopping one's activity.

Physical exercise is the most common factor provoking angina, and patients often become aware of angina for the first time when walking up a hill, or in a hurry. Pain is more likely to occur after a meal, or in cold weather. Some people have angina only in the winter months, with complete clearing during warm weather. Activity following meals, particularly heavy meals, is likely to produce symptoms and some sedentary individuals have angina only after meals. (3)

Intense emotion is likely to produce angina. Anger, anxiety, worry, hurry, sexual activity, public speaking, car driving, and watching competitive sports are all known to be likely to produce angina. Many patients report angina immediately after going to bed (maybe because of cold sheets), and may be awakened by it during the night, particularly following nightmares. (3)

Symptoms seem to vary with the time of day, more than from day to day. Activities such as combing the hair, which require the patient to lift his hands to or above the head level may produce symptoms, while more strenuous activity not requiring elevation of the arms produces none. (2) In the early morning, symptoms are common, and the patient may not be able to shave and prepare for work without stopping, but later in the day may perform moderately heavy labor without discomfort.

Tasks which are routine, which the patient has done for years, may cause no problem, with unfamiliar tasks requiring comparable effort producing symptoms.

The discomfort of angina generally lasts only two or three minutes. If induced by physical activity it diminishes with cessation or slowing of activity; when produced by emotions it subsides more slowly (1) and may last 5 to 15 minutes.

TREATMENT

1. A program of gradually increasing exercise should be encouraged. (1) Patients should begin by exercising to tolerance daily, gradually increasing the amount of exercise as tolerated. When symptoms appear, slow down but do not stop activity. If pain does not diminish or subside, stop until it does.

2. Smoking induces angina in some people and should be avoided. (3) Ten heavy smokers with typical symptoms of angina were exercised until they manifested the first symptoms of angina. Each one performed the test four times while in a non-smoking state, and again four times after smoking. All of the patients developed angina sooner if they had smoked prior to exercise. The average shortening of the exercise period after smoking was 24%. (4)

3. Patients should be careful to keep properly clothed so as not to become chilled. Exposure to cold weather, particularly cold wind on the face, may produce symptoms.

4. Cold drinks may produce symptoms and should be avoided. (3)

5. Begin a weight reduction program if overweight.

6. Use small meals which are easily digested. Never overeat.

7. Eliminate all free fats (oils or grease added to foods; margarine, or mayonnaise) from the diet. Fourteen patients were given a fatty meal and six of them suffered a total of fourteen attacks of angina while at rest during a period of three to five hours after the meal. It was noted that the blood fats were at their peak. (5)

8. Angina at night may be relieved by elevating the head of the bed. Eight of ten patients in a study group had no angina pain at all during the test period. (6)

9. Use a diet free of animal products (vegan diet). A group of four patients were placed on a carefully controlled diet. The first patient had such severe angina he had to stop every nine or ten paces while walking. He was placed on the vegan diet in February, and in August of that year climbed mountains with no angina pain. Patient Number Two had severe angina after walking for five minutes. On the diet he had improvement, and was doing gardening and fairly heavy work without pain, with a normal ECG. After nine months on the diet he gave it up and could not be persuaded to continue. Angina returned with the addition of animal products to his diet. The third patient, after three years on the vegan diet, could climb 2,000 feet up a steep mountain without pain or shortness of breath. The fourth patient, after three to four months on a vegan diet could do heavy work without angina. (7)

APHTHOUS ULCERS

Aphthous ulcers, or canker sores, are oval or round white ulcers surrounded by an area of redness. The Greek word "aphthae" means "to set on fire." They are most commonly found on the cheek, tongue, inner lips, and gums. (8)

The cause is unknown, although viral infections, allergies, stress, vitamin deficiencies, and endocrine imbalance have all been considered. (9) They may occur in up to 40% of the population. Offspring of parents with aphthous ulcers are at a greater risk of developing them. They generally appear by twenty years of age, and are of equal frequency in males and females. As one grows older there is a tendency to have fewer and milder attacks. They heal spontaneously in from one to two weeks (9) but some people are never free of them;

as one heals, others occur. (10) They may appear singly or in crops. (11)

TREATMENT

1. Carefully avoid physical damage to the lining of the mouth. Use a soft toothbrush with no toothpaste, be careful with sharp instruments in the mouth, and avoid sharp foods such as peanut brittle, nuts, etc. Avoid biting the tongue or cheek. Don't talk while chewing, and avoid turning the head to the side while chewing as this tends to promote accidental biting of the tongue.

2. Bland mouth washes such as plain water or saline may be helpful.

3. Vaccines and antibiotics have not proved beneficial (10) and may be harmful. Silver nitrate and chromic acid may give temporary relief, but may delay healing, enlarge the ulcers, and cause scarring. (8)

4. Do not smoke.

5. Be careful with hydration. Drink enough water to keep the urine pale at all times.

6. Eliminate the most common food allergens from the diet (see Appendix A). Fifty-six percent of a group of people studied for food allergies had a history of aphthous ulcers. (12)

7. Alcoholic beverages, chocolate, chewing gum, lozenges, mouthwashes, toothpaste, and sharp, highly seasoned or tart foods, especially citrus fruits should be avoided. (13)

8. Goldenseal powder or a moistened goldenseal tea bag applied directly to the ulcer is one of the best treatments, and may bring rapid relief of pain.

9. A ten minute mouthwash with plain hot water may relieve pain.

ARTHRITIS

Arthritis is an inflammatory or degenerative disease of the joints. The most common forms of arthritis are rheumatoid, osteoarthritis, and gout. (See sections on rheumatoid arthritis and gout.)

TREATMENT

1. Dr. Norman Childers, professor emeritus of horticulture at Rutgers University, has reported that a number of arthritics are

sensitive to the nightshades (eggplant, tomato, white potato, pepper, and tobacco). One study revealed that 87% of arthritics received benefit from a nightshade free diet. (471) Dr. Childers cautions that the diet must be strict; even bits of nightshades are sufficient to nullify the effect of the diet. Foods listing "natural flavoring" as an ingredient may include nightshades. Some yogurts contain potato starch as a thickener. Some cheeses, particularly the pinkish colored ones, may contain paprika. Herbal teas may contain capsicum (pepper). Baby foods may contain potato and tomato products. We suggest a simple diet, free from commercially prepared foods, to eliminate the possibility of unknowingly consuming nightshades. Dr. Childers also reports that chocolate, vitamin C supplements, cortisone or gold shots, tea and coffee may also cause problems. (472)

2. Milk, wheat, egg, corn, and pork have been shown to produce arthritic symptoms. (473) Dr. Breneman states that joint pains are a late manifestation of food allergy, and may not appear for 48 to 72 hours after consumption of the food. Joint pains may not appear for five days after pork consumption. The delay makes it difficult to determine the food causing the problem.

   The allergic reaction causes a temporary accumulation of edema fluid in and around the joint. If the offending foods are not identified and eliminated from the diet permanent deformities occur. Reducing salt intake may decrease fluid retention and relieve discomfort. Alcohol in any form worsens allergic reactions to food.

3. Eating 12 raw pecans a day has been reported to ease some cases of arthritis of the shoulders, arms, and hands in 6 weeks.

4. Sleeping in a sleeping bag often produces a reduction in morning stiffness and pain. (474) An electric blanket may be helpful but is reported less effective.

5. An arthritis liniment may be made by mixing 1 pint alcohol, 1/4 ounce menthol, and 1/2 ounce camphor. Rub on afflicted joints twice daily. Another liniment may be made of equal amounts of mineral oil and alcohol. One tablespoon of oil of wintergreen may be added to each quart of liniment if desired.

6. Overweight increases strain on the joints. The weight should be slightly below average.

7. Hot packs applied to stiff joints often decrease morning stiffness. (475)

8. Avoid immunizations. Arthritis is a relatively frequent complication of rubella (German measles) vaccine in adolescent girls and young women. Various other immunizations have been associated with arthritis. (476)

9. A high protein diet induced arthritis in experimental studies on pigs. Within a week after the start of the diet they demonstrated disturbances of movement and swollen joints. (477)

10. Indole and skatole produced chronic arthritis and extensive joint changes in a group of rabbits. These substances are found in cheese. (534)

11. Contrast baths are often useful in arthritis. Fill one basin with hot water (110-115 degrees F.) and another with cold water (55-60 degrees F.). Immerse the afflicted joint in the hot water for four minutes, then in the cold water for 45 seconds. Alternate back and forth for 20 to 45 minutes. Add hot or cold water as necessary to maintain temperature. In arthritis always begin and end with hot water.

12. Patients unable to exercise joints because of pain may be able to carry out an exercise program in a tub of warm water (93 to 98 degrees F.).

13. Charcoal poultices may be applied to affected joints.

14. A paraffin dip is often soothing. See section on rheumatoid arthritis for procedure.

15. Exercises play a key role in the treatment of arthritis. Refer to the section on rheumatoid arthritis for further suggestions.

Perform each of the following exercises smoothly and slowly five to ten times twice a day. Too little exercise limits joint motion and may cause development of deformities, but too much exercise may aggravate arthritis.

A. Hand and Wrist Exercises

1. Make a fist, then straighten the fingers. If it is difficult to straighten fingers entirely, rest the hand palm down on a table. With the other hand apply pressure to the back of the hand while raising the affected forearm.

2. Spread fingers apart. Touch the tip of each finger to the tip of the thumb, making as round a circle with the fingers as possible.

3. Bend the wrist forward, then around in a circle.

B. Elbow Exercises

    1. Rest the upper arm on a bed or table. Bend elbow to bring the fingers to the shoulders, then straighten arm. Carry out this exercise with the palm turned upward.

C. Shoulder Exercises

    1. Sit in a straight chair with arms resting at the side, palms toward the body. Raise arms sideways, forward, and backward as far as they will go. Raise them up as far as possible.

    2. Standing, bend forward until the top of the body is parallel to the floor. Bracing one hand against the back of a chair may be helpful. Swing the loose arm in circles, making as large an arc as possible.

D. Ankle Exercises

    1. Slowly bend feet up and down, then in and out as far as possible.

    2. Move feet through a circular motion.

E. Knee Exercises

    1. Lie on your back on a firm surface, with legs straight. Contract muscles of the whole leg, flattening knee down on the firm surface. Raise the legs and move them as you would to ride a bicycle.

    2. Sitting on a table or other surface high enough to allow legs to dangle, alternately straighten and bend the knees.

F. Hip Exercises

    1. Lying on the back move the right leg as far to right as possible. Return to starting position and repeat with left leg.

    2. Slowly raise and lower legs with knee straightened, then with knees bent.

    3. Lying face down, lift legs up, keeping knees straight.

G. Neck Exercises

    1. Rotate head in a circle without moving shoulders. Attempt to touch head to each shoulder.

    2. Lying on the back, push the head against the bed as firmly as possible. Lift head up.

H. Back Exercises

1. Lie face down. Tighten hip muscles, hold for a few seconds, then relax. Raise legs keeping knees straight. Place hands on hips, raise head and shoulders and hold two to three seconds. Raise legs and head simultaneously. Place fingers behind head, raise legs with knees straight.

2. Turn over on back. Tighten hip and abdominal muscles to flatten lower back. Raise one leg with knee straight, lower slowly. Repeat with other leg. Raise both legs simultaneously. Raise head and shoulders and lower slowly. Bend one leg, clasp knee with both hands, pulling thigh against abdomen. Relax and repeat with other leg. Repeat the procedure with both legs at the same time.

ASTHMA

Asthma is characterized by wheezing, cough and difficulty breathing. There are two types of asthma: extrinsic and intrinsic. Intrinsic asthma, the more severe, has an allergic cause that cannot be identified. Intrinsic asthma usually develops after the age of 30, and tends to be perennial. (10) Extrinsic asthma generally begins in childhood, is seasonal, and usually is associated with a well-defined history of allergy to a variety of substances.

Four percent (approximately six to eight million) (61) of Americans suffer from asthma. Over half of them are diagnosed between the age of 2 and 17 years; about one-third are initially diagnosed after 30 years of age. Asthma is the leading cause of disease and disability in the 2 to 17 year old group. (10)

Asthma usually begins as a non-productive cough and wheezing; often followed by difficulty breathing and tightness in the chest. Attacks are common during sleep and at night. They generally subside spontaneously in a few hours. (10)

Air passes into and out of the lungs through the trachea, which branches out into the right and left bronchus. The bronchi branch tree-like out into smaller air passages. The smallest passages are called bronchi and bornchioles. A muscular wall constricts or opens the bronchi and bronchioles. When the wall is open air moves freely in and out of the small air sacs called alveoli which are found at the end of the bronchioles. Effective respiration takes place in the alveoli; when the muscular walls of the bronchiole constrict it is difficult for air to pass freely, and air tends to become trapped in the sacs. Forcing air out through the narrow airway produces the wheezing sound. The lining of the bronchi may become inflamed and swollen, and thick mucus tends to collect. The oxygen level in the blood may fall, producing cyanosis (bluish discoloration).

Most asthmatics have an allergic disorder, (62) but some, perhaps 20%, may not.

TREATMENT OF ACUTE ATTACKS

1. Pouring cold water on the back of the neck is helpful in controlling asthma. (48) The patient bends over and cold water is poured on the back of the neck from a pitcher holding about a gallon of water held about 24 inches above the neck for 30 to 90 seconds. The treatment is repeated 2-3 times daily.

2. Fever therapy was helpful in over half of a group of patients given four treatments on a weekly basis. Body temperature was raised to 104 to 105 degrees F. and kept there for five to seven hours. The first or second treatment often brought relief. (49) Another researcher successfully used a course of two to four treatments each of three hours duration, raising the temperature to between 102 and 105 degrees F. (50)

3. A number of asthmatic medications contain sodium metabisulfite and should be avoided. A 23-year-old asthmatic was hospitalized five times during a six month period. She was given intravenous medication for her asthma and about one hour later she rapidly grew worse, requiring assisted ventilation and intubation. Her physicians began to suspect a sensitivity to metabisulfite and tests proved positive. After six months free of tartrazine, sodium benzoate, and sodium metabisulfite she was able to control her asthma without the use of steroids. Unfortunately most of the drugs that contain metasulfite do not identify it on the label or the literature. (57) Avoid drugs if at all possible. Corticosteroids are often used. Long-term corticosteroid therapy may decrease resistance to infection, impair wound healing, raise blood pressure, induce weight gain, ulcers, muscle weakness, diabetes, cataracts, fluid retention, skin problems, loss of potassium, increase the likelihood of bone fractures, menstrual problems, mental disturbances, and impaired growth in children. (10, 63)

4. Hot fomentations to the back of the neck and thorax and front of the chest are helpful, along with a hot foot bath. Keep the head cool by sponging with cool water or use a fan. The treatment

should be continued until the attack subsides, generally within 15 to 30 minutes. Finish off with a shower or alchol rub. Rest in bed until sweating subsides.

5. A cool air vaporizer may be used during an acute attack. Menthol or oil of eucalyptus may be used if desired.

6. Garlic has been used for hundreds of years in the treatment of asthma. Blend one clove of garlic in one cup of hot water. Some patients vomit after drinking the solution and this assists in loosening bronchial secretions. Give a second cup if the first is vomited, as the active ingredient is excreted through the lungs after intestinal absorption.

7. A cup of hot water, mullein, or catnip tea may be given each hour.

8. Some find a neutral bath (94-97 degrees F.) helpful. Patients may remain in the tub for up to two hours.

9. Aerosol nebulizers have been shown to produce a rebound similar to that produced by nosedrops, forcing the patient to use more and more medication while obtaining less and less relief. Some authorities in the field of asthma are discontinuing the use of this type of medication. These medications may also dry the secretions in the lungs, producing thick mucus plugs. There is also the possibility that these medications will interact with other medications, producing what could be a fatal heart irregularity. (64)

MAINTENANCE THERAPY

Asthmatics should be encouraged to have a program of regular physical exercise. Brief exercise periods of from one to two minutes can actually open up constricted lungs according to a report from the Committee on Rehabilitation Therapy of the American Academy of Allergy. (65) The asthmatic should select sports that involve only short periods of sporadic effort. Baseball and swimming (in warm water 85 to 90 degrees F.) are apparently excellent forms of exercise for asthmatics. (66)

Dr. Arend Bouhuys of Emory University in Atlanta, Georgia, recommends that asthma sufferers learn to play a wind instrument or sing to improve their breathing capacity. A person at rest uses only about 10% of his lung capacity; hard work increases lung use only to about 50%. The singer or woodwind player uses his lungs almost to the fullest extent possible. (67)

1. Breathing exercises:

Each exercise should be performed five or six times twice a day, and at the first sign of an attack.

A. To achieve full anterior expansion stand tall with hands on shoulders, elbows together in front of you. As you breathe in, stretch your elbows back, and bring them together again as you breathe out.

B. Maximal lateral rib expansion is achieved by standing straight, one arm at your side, and the other curled over your head. As you breathe in slide the hand beside you down the side of your leg, and back up as you breathe out. Reverse arm position and repeat.

C. Standing tall with shoulders back and breathing deeply will develop proper breathing techniques.

D. Ventral stretch and lifting of the rib cage may be achieved by kneeling so you sit on your legs. While breathing in, stretch both hands up as you come up on your knees; breathe out while kneeling back on your legs and lowering arms.

E. Lying on your stomach, clasp your hands together over your hips. Lift your head and shoulders while breathing in, relax as you breathe out.

F. Turn over on your back, with your arms above your head. Breathe in as you lift both legs; lower them as you breathe out. This gives abdominal muscle control.

G. Still lying on your back, bend your knees up. Lift your hips off the floor as you breathe in. Lower them as you breathe out.

H. Lie on your back with arms at your side, and your feet slightly apart. Breathe in as you lift your arms up and back over your head; breathe out as you sit up to touch your toes. Breathe in while lying back and breathe out as you relax.

I. For ten minutes, and at the first sign of an asthmatic attack, sit up straight in a chair. Inhale through your nose and exhale through pursed lips. Pursing the lips assists in opening the bronchial tubes. (69)

J. Postural drainage will assist in clearing the mucus from the lungs. Lie on your stomach, with your head and chest draped over the edge of your bed. Bring up the sputum by coughing gently for 2-3 minutes. During an attack some people cannot tolerate this position, and they may lie face down in bed with two or three pillows under their hips. (69)

    K. Lie flat on the bed with knees bent. Slowly raise the right knee to the chest while breathing out and tensing the abdominal muscles; lower the right leg, inhale, and relax abdominal muscles. Repeat procedure with the left leg. (70)

2. Avoid the use of synthetic fabrics. Apparently dust collects on synthetic fabrics because of the static electricity generated by friction and motion. Static electricity develops most readily in dry material and a dry atmosphere. Cotton and wool, natural fibers, attract and hold moisture, while synthetic fibers do not; therefore synthetic fibers are more readily charged with static electricity. (51)

3. Use of a diet free of cereals, milk, eggs, chocolate, fish, and other common allergenic foods enabled a group of 50 children and 45 adults to relieve their asthma without the use of vaccines, antigens, ACTH or corticosteroids. The diet must be adhered to strictly. (52) The author of the report states that skin test studies often fail to identify the foods responsible.

4. Avoid the use of foods containing additives, tartrazine (a yellow food dye) acetylsalicylic acid, sulfur-dioxide, and sodium benzoate which are all known to provoke asthma in sensitive individuals. (53) Sodium metabisulfite, found in fruit juices, alcoholic beverages, vinegar, processed meats, dehydrated vegetables, processed cheeses, syrups and toppings, causes asthma in some people. (57)

5. Live in the country, in an area of minimal air pollution. Sulfur dioxide may produce an immediate increase in airway resistance in even normal persons, and one study revealed an increased number of asthmatic attacks during times of high atmospheric pollution. (54)

6. Make it a practice to breathe through the nose rather than the mouth. Approximately 90% of asthmatics are mouth breathers. (55) Organisms in the mouth and throat are more readily transmitted to the lungs in mouth breathers, increasing the incidence of respiratory tract infections. Mouth breathing also brings cold air into the trachea which may result in wheezing. Allergenic particles may penetrate further into the respiratory system with mouth breathing.

7. Sleep on your stomach. This aids in natural drainage, removing secretions and infection from the lungs as well as encouraging the mouth to remain closed.

8. Many patients can stop wheezing by the use of "sleep breathing." (55) Sleep breathing is slower and deeper than usual, with a three second pause at the top of the inspiration and at the end of the expiration. Patients should learn to sleep breathe at all times. (55)

9. Camomile tea has an antiallergic action. Drink one cup morning and evening. (71)

10. Avoid bananas and melons as many asthmatics are sensitive to them, particularly those who are also sensitive to ragweed. (56)

11. Sleep outdoors if possible. This is more beneficial than sleeping in a room with the windows and doors open. (58)

12. Antihistamines have little effect on the source of asthma and should not be used. Apparently histamine is not a major factor in the allergic reaction. (59)

13. Dead, decomposed cockroaches were found to be the cause of asthma in approximately 40% of patients allergic to housedust. (60)

14. Avoid fumes and strong odors such as turpentine, gasoline, paints, various chemicals, heavily scented flowers, perfumes, etc. (61)

15. Chilling, cold air, and sudden barometric changes may precipitate an attack. (61) Dress to prevent chilling, being particularly careful to keep the limbs well clothed.

16. Drink sufficient water to stay well hydrated, and keep secretions from thickening. (61) Hot garlic tea (see Cystitis section) helps some.

17. Avoid crowds and other sources of infection. (61)

18. Many asthmatics are sensitive to animal dander. House pets should be excluded. (61)

19. House plants may contain mold spores and should be eliminated. (61) Guard against mold in bathrooms, etc. Scrupulous cleanliness is mandatory.

20. Many asthmatics are allergic to nuts, shellfish, tomatoes, strawberries, house dusts, feathers, and furniture stuffing. Drugs such as vaccines, penicillin, aspirin, and anesthetic agents may all precipitate asthmatic attacks. Pollen from trees, grasses, and weeds are notorious in asthma.

21. Do not smoke or be around people who smoke. Nonsmokers in the presence of smokers have been shown to suffer some of the same ill-effects as do the smokers. Children whose mothers smoke are at increased risk of developing asthma. As much as 34% of childhood asthma may be due to parental smoking. (72)

22. Some people are allergic to chicle, the base of chewing gum. (73)

23. Infants should be breast-fed. Infants born to allergic mothers and fed cow's milk have a greater incidence of asthma than infants with similar histories but who were breast-fed. Cat dander and egg were the most common allergens in either breast or bottle-fed infants. That cow's milk may cause a flare-up of asthma has been suspected for many years. Because allergens may be transmitted through breast milk, breast-feeding mothers should avoid the use of milk and eggs. (74)

24. A 1953 medical journal reported the successful treatment of asthma with a fat-free diet. (75) See Appendix C.

25. Efforts should be made to eliminate dust from the home. Plain, simple furniture designs catch less dust than ornate furniture. Fabric upholstery should be eliminated and plastic or rubberized canvas used in its place. Open bookshelves and books are dust catchers. All clothing should be kept in closets and never allowed to lie about the room. Closet doors should be kept closed. Wool clothing should be kept in zippered bags. Avoid moth-balls, insect sprays, tar paper, and camphor. Flooring should be linoleum or wood, with no rugs of any kind. Toys should be wood, metal, or plastic; no stuffed toys. Avoid cosmetics, talc, perfumes, and flowers in the room. Walls should be painted or papered with washable wallpaper. Pictures and other dust catchers should be removed. Washable cotton or synthetic window shades should be used. No venetian blinds. Washable cotton or fiberglass curtains may be used, but no draperies. Air conditioning is helpful. Electric fans stir up dust and should not be used. Synthetics such as dacron should be used for pillows. Kapok, feathers, and foam rubber are not satisfactory. Non-fuzzy washable cotton or synthetic blankets may be used. Use a washable cotton bed-spread rather than chenille. Pillows, mattress, and box springs should be covered with allergen-proof encasings. Zippered plastic covers are not adequate to seal out dust. The room should be wet-dusted twice a day. A disinfectant may be used to damp mop the floor to prevent the growth of mold spores. (61) Forced hot air heating systems used in the winter

tend to blow molds and dust around the house. An air filtration system may be helpful.

26. Abdominal breathing should be practiced at all times. Abdominal breathing is accomplished mainly by diaphragmatic excursion and involves some movement of the lower intercostals. It can account for 60% of the vital capacity and is much more efficient than thoracic breathing as it literally pushes air in and out of the bases of the lungs. Thoracic breathing is done by the intercostal muscles and is often seen in women whose girdles and corsets have changed their breathing habits. (76) Good posture encourages abdominal breathing and should be practiced at all times.

27. In a study of 1,674 children hospitalized before the age of two years, 13% of them showed later asthma, as compared to 5% for the non-hospitalized group. Children admitted during the first year of life had a 14-16% chance of developing bronchitis, compared to 7% of the non-hospitalized group. (529)

28. Anise tea is especially helpful in bronchial asthma attacks. (307)

29. Exhaling forcefully through a small drinking straw into a large bottle of water forces expansion of the spastic bronchial tubes and may relieve an asthmatic attack. (273)

30. People who have hay fever, asthma, or a respiratory infection should avoid the use of hair sprays. Dr. Donald Schlueter of the Medical College of Wisconsin at Milwaukee feels that the perfume in the hair sprays causes reactions. He suggests that people using hair spray try to hold their breath while spraying. Sprays should be used only in well-ventilated areas and users should leave the area immediately after spraying. (546)

ATHLETE'S FOOT

Athlete's foot, also called Tinea pedis, and ringworm of the feet, is the most common superficial fungus infection. (34) It is uncommon in areas of the world where the people never wear shoes.

TREATMENT

1. Use one of the following solutions as a 20 to 30 minute foot bath twice a day.

   A. Four ounces of thyme to a pint of alcohol. (35)

B. Goldenseal tea. After drying, dust with goldenseal powder.

C. Sea water or saline made with sea salt.

D. One clove of garlic blended in one quart of water.

2. Wash the feet, particularly the area between the toes, with soap and water, and dry carefully twice a day. Put on clean socks.

3. Use socks that allow the evaporation of moisture. Canvas sneakers or sandals are best. Avoid shoes with plastic linings. Change shoes every other day to allow moisture to escape.

4. Small pieces of cotton placed between the toes at night will help absorb moisture.

5. Use white cotton socks. (36) Cotton absorbs perspiration better than synthetic materials. Coloring dyes may produce an allergic reaction, further complicating the problem.

6. Expose the feet to sunshine at least 10 to 15 minutes a day.

7. Do not walk barefoot around swimming pools and public places.

8. Apple cider vinegar (or any vinegar) has been reported useful. Apply every time itching begins, and after every bath to stop fungus growth.

9. Rub the infected area with a cut clove of garlic.

10. Cornstarch dusted on the feet will help control moisture.

11. Cotton balls may be soaked in honey and placed between the toes at bedtime. Cover feet with socks to keep the bed clean.

12. Hot and cold foot baths may be used. Fill a foot tub with enough hot water to come up above the ankles. The water should be as hot as can be tolerated, and more hot water should be added as the foot-bath cools. Keep the feet in hot water for six minutes, then use a one minute ice water soak. Repeat the hot and cold three times. Dry feet thoroughly, and dust with cornstarch or goldenseal powder. The treatment may be repeated every two hours in severe cases.

13. Avoid the use of athlete's foot remedies commonly obtained from the drug store. In one study 40% of the people using the products were found to be allergic to one or more of the ingredients. Boric acid is readily absorbed into the body where the skin is broken and may produce toxicity. It is found in many over-the-counter athlete's foot remedies. (37, 38)

14. Griseofulvin is often prescribed for stubborn cases of athlete's foot, but studies have shown that this medicine produces cancer

in mice. "To demonstrate that griseofulvin is not a carcinogen in man would ... require at least a 20-year follow-up of griseofulvin-treated patients, comparing the incidence of malignant tumors to the incidence in a comparable group of control patients. There are no such data." (39) It is toxic to the offspring and should never be given to pregnant women. More immediate side-effects of griseofulvin include headache, mental confusion, blood dyscrasias, and gastrointestinal disturbances.

BACKACHE

Most Americans suffer from backache at some time during their life. Our lifestyle is sedentary, predisposing to weak muscles and overweight.

TREATMENT

1. Exercise is invaluable in the treatment of low back pain. The following exercises should be done 6 to 10 times each at the beginning of the program and gradually increased until 15 to 25 are done at each session. (395, 396)

   A. Lie on the back on a firm surface with a pillow under the head. Bend the knees with the feet at least 12 inches apart. Straighten arms, pointing fingers toward the ceiling. Sit up smoothly, and attempt to touch the floor between the knees with the fingertips. Lower the body to the lying position, and repeat the exercise. This exercise causes contraction of the abdominal muscles.

   B. Still in the lying position of exercise A, move the feet closer together. Tighten the muscles of the hips, lifting the hips as far off the floor as possible. Hold the position for a second, then relax slowly, easing back down into the original position. Repeat. This exercise strengthens the hip muscles. Do not raise the back off the floor above the waistline as this will cause the back to arch.

   C. Bring your knees up until you can grasp them below the kneecaps, one knee in each hand. Separate the legs 15 to 18 inches and pull the knees as close to the armpits as possible. Pull both knees at the same time. Relax to allow the arms to extend, but do not let go of the knees. Repeat the pulling process. This exercise is designed to straighten the strong, short back muscles. Many people find this exercise brings more pain relief than any other, and some report that they do this exercise first as the remainder of the exercises can then be performed with less discomfort.

D. Sit on the floor with the legs extended and straight in front of you. Bend slowly and smoothly forward, trying to touch the toes. Sit up straight and repeat. This exercise stretches the back muscles and helps restore and maintain a full range of forward movement of the low back. If you have pain in the leg do not do this exercise as it stretches the sciatic nerve and increases the pain. When the pain is gone the exercise should be begun promptly.

E. Stand comfortably, with all muscles relaxed. Place the right foot 6 to 10 inches behind and slightly to the right of the left foot. Lower the body to a squatting position while keeping the left foot constantly flat on the floor. Straighten the arms and place both palms flat on the floor. Stretch the right leg as far as possible to the rear, placing the toes turned slightly to the left in such a way that they will act as a spring. Lift the hips and thrust downward, keeping the right leg straight. Bring the right leg up beside the left, putting the foot flat on the floor. Extend the left leg to the rear, and repeat the exercise. Draw the left leg in until the foot is 6 to 10 inches behind and slightly to the left of the right foot, firmly contract the hip muscles and return to the standing position. Do not raise the hips ahead of the rest of the body as this will shift the strain to the back muscles. While one of the most complex and physically difficult of the exercises, this is also one of the most effective.

F. Stand relaxed with the feet about 18 inches apart, toes pointed straight ahead. Point the fingers to a location about 12 inches in front of your feet, and squat to touch that location. The feet must be kept flat on the floor. Return to standing position and repeat.

2. One physician reported complete relief of low back pain by sleeping in a hammock. (397)

3. A foot exercise has been helpful in low back pain. Dr. Walter Meyers at the Veterans Medical Center in Hot Springs, South Dakota, reports gratifying results with this simple exercise: The patient lies flat on a firm surface and flexes his feet alternately up and down. He then alternately flexes and relaxes the hip muscles in coordination with the foot flexion. The exercise is

continued until the patient has muscle fatigue and is repeated four to six times a day. (398)

4. Smoking has been linked to low back pain. Dr. John W. Frymoyer, a professor of orthopedics and rehabilitation at the University of Vermont observed that 53% of a group of patients with severe back pain had smoked at least a pack-and-a-half a day for 19 pack years; 47% of the back pain patients were non-smokers. In a pain-free control group, 60% were non-smokers, and 40% had smoked less than a pack a day for 14 pack-years. Dr. Frymoyer states that there is a definite relationship between smoker's cough and severe back pain. Dr. Frymoyer found that injecting the nicotine equivalent of one cigarette significantly reduced the measured blood flow in the vertebral body. Dr. Vert Mooney, chairman of orthopedics at the University of Texas at Dallas says that smoking may interfere with the elasticity of connective tissue. (399)

5. Dr. Gerald Hirschberg, Clinical Professor of Physical Medicine and Rehabilitation at the University of California College of Medicine says that 20% of low back pain may be linked to flat feet. He suggests that patients with low back pain check for flat feet by wetting their feet and placing them on material such as brown paper which will show a clear print. If the print is solid, without indentation along the big toe side of the foot, the foot is flat. Treatment consists of an arch support or inlay inside the shoe. (400)

6. Muscle strain is the most common cause of back pain. Rest in bed for 24 hours is generally the only treatment required. The bed should be firm to keep the spine straight. A 1/2 to 3/4 inch thick bedboard may be placed between the mattress and box springs to support the back. Place 1 or 2 pillows under the knees to straighten the lumbar curve. When lying on the side flex the knees and place the pillow between them. Avoid sleeping on the stomach as it increases swayback and twists the neck. The body is heavier than the shoulders or legs, and sags into the bed, arching the back.

7. When sitting, use a straight chair with a firm back. The knees should be higher than the hips. A small footstool may be required. Avoid overstuffed chairs and sofas. Do not sit in the same position for long periods without getting up and moving around. Chair arms support the shoulders and upper back.

8. When driving, push the car seat forward to raise the knees

higher than the hips. This reduces strain on the back and shoulder muscles. Always use safety belts.

9. Don't stand in the same position for long periods of time. Shift the weight from one foot to another. When doing such things as ironing, place one foot on a footstool to reduce swayback.

10. Women should wear low-heeled shoes most of the time. Heels higher than about one inch should not be worn more than four hours per week.

11. Lift with the legs, not the back. Squat in front of the object to be lifted. Holding it close to your body rise slowly to the standing position. Do not lift from a bending forward position as occurs when reaching over furniture to open and close windows. Don't lift heavy objects from car trunks.

12. Exercise out-of-doors daily. Warm up gradually to prevent ligament strain.

13. Wear clothing adequate to prevent chilling of the body when perspiring. Do not go into air conditioning when perspiring.

14. Soaking in a tub of warm water may be quite relaxing to a strained back. Before doing heavy exercise avoid using water that is too hot, as it relaxes the muscles, and may leave them more susceptible to injury.

15. Constantly aim for good posture.

16. Being overweight places an additional burden on the muscles. Reduce if you are overweight.

17. During the first 72 hours after a back strain an eight minute ice massage may be very effective. Use ice cubes or a block of ice made by freezing water in a paper cup or frozen fruit juice can. Massage the painful area and about six inches surrounding it. After 72 hours use alternating hot and cold. Wring a towel out of hot water and apply for 30 seconds, with four or five alterations. "Applying an ice pack will often do more to relieve muscle spasm than any medication." (401) Moist heat reduces local inflammation and increases local blood flow.

BAD BREATH

Bad breath, or halitosis, is a problem of great concern to many Americans. The word "halitosis" comes from the Latin "halitus" (breath) and the Greek suffix "osis" (condition or pathologic process).

There are many causes of bad breath, but with careful study of the problem the cause can usually be determined.

TREATMENT

1. Dehydration is a primary cause of bad breath. Drink enough water to keep the urine pale at all times. Early morning halitosis is often caused by dehydration. There is no flow of saliva during sleep, which allows putrefaction of the oral epithelial cells which have flaked off, but not been removed by the flow of saliva.

2. Disorders of the oral cavity are felt to cause 56 to 85% of all cases of bad breath. (289) Poor oral hygiene, plaque, caries, gingivitis, stomatitis, periodontitis, "hairy tongue," and oral carcinoma have all been known to cause bad breath. Proper dental care, frequent flossing and brushing of the teeth, and brushing of the tongue are adequate to control bad breath in most cases. The American Council on Dental Therapeutics believes that mouthwash does not substantially contribute to oral health (289) and the Food and Drug Administration has required the manufacturers of nine brands of mouthwash to stop using advertisements claiming that their product is effective in destroying the bacteria that cause bad breath. Toothpaste is pleasant to use, but not necessary in oral hygiene.

3. Breathing through the mouth causes bad breath by decreasing the amount of saliva due to evaporation. Such conditions as enlarged adenoids, nasal infection, hay fever, and a deviated nasal septum encourage mouth breathing.

4. A foul-smelling discharge associated with sinusitis may cause bad breath. Treating the sinusitis will cure the bad breath. Adenoiditis, pulmonary abscess, bronchiectsis, empyema, peritonsillar abscess, tonsillitis, etc., and numerous systemic diseases may also induce bad breath.

5. Brush the tongue carefully. The tongue is often coated with food particles or debris and should be cleaned.

6. If you suspect that you have bad breath you may use a simple test. Touch the back of your hand with your tongue and smell the hand. The odor will give you the answer. Another test is to

cover the mouth and nose with both hands and exhale strongly, smelling the breath.

7. Detergent foods such as apples, carrots, celery, etc., help in cleansing the teeth and removing odor-causing bacteria from the mouth.

8. Some people believe that outdoor exercise, such as walking, brings more oxygen into the lungs, diluting and removing odorous substances in the system and decreasing bad breath.

9. Halitosis has also been called "heavy breath." Reports of food allergies inducing heavy breath have appeared in the medical literature. (289, 290) A trial period of elimination of the most common allergy-producing foods (See Appendix A) may be worthwhile.

10. "The therapy of true halitosis lies in reducing in the diet the intake of fatty aromatic substances, particularly the milk or butter fats . . ." (292, 291)

11. Avoiding constipation will help bad breath.

12. Taking charcoal by mouth will assist with bad breath caused by constipation or oral factors. Let the charcoal tablet dissolve slowly in the mouth.

13. Thyme tea may be quite helpful in cases of bad breath caused by gastric disturbances. (301)

BEDWETTING

Bedwetting, or enuresis, is a problem all too common to parents. At the age of two, 50% of children wet the bed at night; by age four the figure drops to 10 to 15%. Less than 5% still wet at age 12. Boys are more troubled with bedwetting than girls, blacks more than whites, and children who were underweight at birth more than those with normal birth weights. (110) Bedwetting in girls predisposes to urinary tract infection; the more frequently they wet the bed the more likely they are to develop a urinary tract infection. (109)

Most bedwetters have a small bladder capacity, and this small capacity makes it difficult for them to go through the night without voiding. Bedwetters pass urine frequently during the day. The bladder is generally normal anatomically; the small size is because the bladder is in spasm, and when the cause of spasm is removed the bladder enlarges. (109)

TREATMENT

1. There is much evidence that the primary cause of bedwetting is allergy. Bedwetting in children is associated with a much higher rate of hay fever, hives, urinary tract infection, and food and drug allergies in both parents. (111)

   A 1978 study of 100 bedwetting children revealed that removing milk from the diet stopped the bedwetting in over half of the children. The investigators felt that milk lowers the voiding reflex threshold by its action on the inhibitory center of the brain stem. (112)

   The American College of Allergists in their 1980 meeting was told that about 5.5 million American children wet the bed each night because of a food allergy. Cow's milk was the offending agent in about 60% of cases; chocolate, eggs, grains and citrus fruits were also incriminated. (116) Removing from the food from the diet brought an almost instant cure to bedwetting. An earlier study revealed that in a group of 60 bedwetters, 24 were sensitive to milk, 20 to wheat, 17 to egg, 13 to corn, 4 to chicken and orange, and smaller numbers to pork, tomato, peanut, beef, apple, fish, berries, peas, chocolate, rye, and cauliflower. (113) One researcher reported success with a diet which also eliminated foods containing salicylates (Appendix B), and foods containing additives (including sugar and honey) in addition to milk and chocolate. (110) Dr. B. Feingold, who is famous for his work with hyperactive children, reports that hyperactive children have a high incidence of bedwetting, and that his diet is often helpful. (110)

2. Constipation may contribute to bedwetting. A large mass of fecal material can decrease bladder capacity. (114)

3. Various exercises have been recommended in the treatment of enuresis. Probably the most common is merely to stop and start the flow of urine each time the child urinates. Some bedwetters will benefit in six weeks, but others may require longer. To train the bladder to hold more urine some authorities suggest that the child put off going to the bathroom as long as possible after they feel the urge.

4. An exercise to reduce pressure on the urinary bladder has been used with success. The bedwetter lies on his back on any hard surface. With arms stretched back of the head, the patient lifts small weights (such as one pound cans of fruits or vegetables) to a vertical position, and lowers them, repeating the

exercise until moderately fatigued. The exercise should be carried out with deep breathing. (115) the same author suggests the "Indian Dance" exercise: bouncing up and down in warm water deep enough to cause a pull on the chest.

5. Since diseases such as pinworms, anemia, upper respiratory tract infections, or any toxic condition may predispose to bedwetting, these should be treated. (115)

6. Many children have a temporary cure of their bedwetting during the summer months when they are out-of-doors and more physically active. The bedwetter should be encouraged to have vigorous exercise out-of-doors daily. (115)

7. In younger children a foot massage may assist in improving muscle tone of the feet, and induce a feeling of well-being in the child. There may be a secondary benefit to the bladder. (115)

8. Many children who have stopped bedwetting have a return of the problem during the winter months. Dress the child warmly when out-of-doors. (110) Chilling increases bladder tone.

BELL'S PALSY

Bell's palsy is a weakness of facial muscles of unknown cause. Viruses are suspect because the disease often follows a respiratory infection. Patients frequently report exposure to drafts or chilling of that portion of the face prior to the onset of Bell's palsy and some feel this is a cause. Still others feel that a lack of blood supply to the involved nerve is the cause.

The disease may be of sudden onset; some patients awaken in the morning with facial paralysis. Others have a pain around the ear and face for a few hours or even days prior to onset of the paralysis. There follows a "drawing" sensation on the affected side of the face, sagging of the upper lip, inability to close the eye on the afflicted side, and inability to wrinkle the forehead. Many have excessive watering of the eyes and difficulty eating and drinking. There may be taste impairment. If the eye is forced closed the eye on the paralyzed side will roll upward (Bell's phenomenon).

All patients with partial palsy, and three-quarters of those with complete palsy recover with no treatment of any kind. In fact, "watchful neglect" is probably the most important treatment. As few as 7% of patients are dissatisfied with the outcome of the disease (503) when handled in this way. Certainly corticosteroids should be avoided. Severe taste impairment and/or reduced tearing of the eyes are bad prognostic signs, particularly in older patients.

Bell's palsy occurs in both males and females and may occur at any age, but most cases occur between 20 and 40 years of age. There may be a genetic predisposition. (504) It is more common in the summer months, particularly in August. About three persons out of 2000 will have Bell's palsy, and approximately 7% of these will have it more than once. Generally the younger the patient the better the chance of recovery.

TREATMENT

1. Most Bell's palsy patients recovery spontaneously and should not be given pharmaceuticals or surgical treatment. (503) The patient often fears he has had a stroke and may need much reassurance and support.

2. Moist heat in the form of warm wet washcloths may be applied twice daily for 20 minutes to relieve pain and tenseness. Follow this with gentle massage backward and upward.

3. After a few days, as muscle tone begins to return, the patient should do facial exercises for five minutes three times a day. Standing in front of a mirror he should wrinkle the forehead, close the affected eye, purse the lips, draw the mouth to one side, blow out the cheeks and try to whistle.

4. Liquid and soft foods may make eating easier. Use small feedings and do not overeat.

5. Adhesive tape may be used to support sagging facial muscles.

6. The eye requires special attention to keep it moist and free from dirt and dust. An artificial tear solution used four times a day will assist in maintaining moisture. Sun glasses will decrease evaporation from the eye by protecting it from the wind. Periodically closing the eyelid with the fingertip will alleviate constant eyestrain. An eyepatch should be used at night. (502)

7. Most authors agree that there is considerable edema of the nerve during the acute phase of the disease. A low salt diet and charcoal compresses worn nightly may encourage removal of this fluid.

8. Chilling and drafts are often associated with the onset of Bell's palsy. Keep the face warm and free from drafts. A draft is a current of air that chills the skin to any degree. Compare the temperature of the forehead with that of the skin to be tested. They should both be the same temperature.

9. Increasing the humidity may increase the patient's comfort.

10. Surgery has been used in the treatment of Bell's palsy, but the results are no better than if surgery is avoided. Exploratory surgery might be indicated, however, to determine the cause if no improvement occurs within a year or two, (503) provided a tumor or other specific disease of the nerve is suspected.

11. Predisone is sometimes given, but there is no proof that it is effective. (505) Because of the very unwanted side-effects, it should not be used.

BRONCHIECTASIS

Bronchiectasis is permanent dilation and infection of one or more bronchi. Chronic cough with sputum is the most prominent symptom. The patient may cough up blood or blood-stained sputum and have inflammation of the lungs. Lying down empties secretions from the lower lobes of the lungs into the bronchi and may induce coughing. (507) Patients with advanced disease may have shortness of breath on exertion. The patient may complain of a general feeling of illness and fatigue.

Pulmonary infections and obstruction of the bronchi, aspiration of foreign bodies, vomitus, etc., and pressure from tumors, enlarged lymph nodes and dilated blood vessels are felt to be causes. (506)

TREATMENT

1. Good hydration is important as it keeps the sputum thinner and easier to expel.

2. Smoking, pollens, fumes, aerosols, and dusts are bronchial irritants and increase secretions. Sweeping and dusting should be avoided unless a good mask is worn.

3. Postural drainage should be done for 20 minutes twice daily.

4. A vaporizer used nightly and constantly in cool, dry air may provide humidification and assist in keeping secretions liquid.

5. Wear a scarf or mask over the mouth and nose to warm air in cold weather. Try to avoid sudden temperature changes. Maintain 30 to 50% humidity for best mucociliary function.

6. Avoid persons with respiratory tract infections. Avoid crowds and poorly ventilated rooms. Begin vigorous treatment at the first sign of any cold.

7. Avoid cough medications and antihistamines as they dry secretions, making them harder to expel.

8. Learn to cough productively. Using diaphragmatic breathing, breathe slowly and deeply. Hold the breath for several seconds, the cough two short, forceful coughs with the mouth open. The first cough loosens the secretions, and the second should remove them. Hold breath for a few seconds, then inhale gently. A vigorous inhalation may induce non-productive coughing.

9. Extremely hot or cold foods may provoke coughing and should be avoided.

10. Gas-forming foods cause abdominal distention, restricting diaphragmatic movement during respiration.

11. Avoid fatigue and any degree of chilling as these lower general resistance and worsen symptoms.

12. Scrupulous oral hygiene is important because of the sputum production. Bacterial growth in the mouth must be discouraged by the use of a soft bristle brush and plenty of rinsing. Avoid mouth washes because of their harshness and ineffectiveness.

13. Tight bands around the abdomen are unhealthful for anyone, and doubly so in bronchiectasis.

BRONCHITIS

Bronchitis is an infection or inflammation of the bronchi, the two main branches of the trachea. They divide into many smaller bronchi like tree roots. Bronchitis may be induced by infections or by chemical or physical agents such as fumes, smoke, dust, etc. (459)

Acute bronchitis generally begins after an upper respiratory infection, with a gradual onset of cough. Wheezing, and acute respiratory distress follow. There may be fever, chilliness, muscle aches, headache, hoarseness, and dry, scratchy throat.

Chronic bronchitis is due to repeated bouts of acute bronchitis, from allergies, or any chronic irritant, especially tobacco smoke.

TREATMENT

1. The chief cause of bronchitis is probably smoking. Only 9% of bronchitis patients in the United States are non-smokers. (460) During the first year of life an infant's risk of bronchitis and pneumonia is doubled by exposure to his parents's cigarette smoke. (461) If both parents smoke risk is higher than if only one smokes. It is lowest if neither parent smokes.

2. Children in homes where gas is used in cooking have a higher incidence of bronchitis than children in homes where electricity is used. (462)

3. Several authorities feel that some bronchitis is due to allergy. Albert Rowe, M.D., reported that food allergy is the sole cause of 25 to 40% of all cases of bronchial asthma. (463) One group of children with recurrent bronchitis were cured of all their symptoms when milk was removed from their diet. (464)

4. Exercise is helpful in chronic bronchitis. A group placed on an exercise program showed significant improvement when compared to a non-exercising control group. (465)

5. Coughing will encourage removal of mucus. Eight patients coughed once a minute for 20 minutes and showed a 41% increase in clearance of mucus from the lungs. (466) Avoid cough suppressants.

6. Anise tea and almond milk have been reported helpful in bronchitis. To make the almond milk blend six tablespoons of almonds in a pint of water. (467)

7. Avoid the use of expectorants as they are of dubious value, and often produce nausea, vomiting, and gastric irritation. (468) Antihistamines and decongestants make it more difficult to eliminate the mucus.

8. A vaporizor may be quite effective in assisting expectoration. An hour of aerosol inhalation of a water mist reduced sputum thickness and made expectoration easier in 20 cases of bronchitis. (469) Oil of eucalyptus may be added to the water if desired. (470)

9. A high fluid intake will assist in keeping the sputum thin so it can be more easily coughed up. Water is the very best expectorant.

10. Moist heat applications to the chest are very effective. Apply a hot towel to the chest for three minutes, cold for thirty seconds, with three to five changes.

11. Hot drinks stimulate productive coughing and relieve congestion.

12. Avoid fatigue and chilling. Walking barefoot across a cold floor is sufficient to prolong symptoms.

13. Deep breathing exercises should be taken three to four times a day. Take a deep breath, hold a few seconds and exhale. Repeat 10 to 20 times.

14. Apply a heating compress at night. Squeeze a thin piece of cotton fabric from cold water, place it against the chest, cover well on all sides with a piece of plastic, and hold in place with long strips of material such as bed sheeting, or a tightfitting sweater.

15. A hot foot bath, acting as a "derivative" will relieve chest congestion.

16. Postural drainage may reduce retention of secretions. See section on asthma for procedure.

BUERGER'S DISEASE

Buerger's disease, also called thromboangiitis obliterans, is an inflammation of the walls of the blood vessels, with clot formation, thickening and scarring of the blood vessel walls, and eventual closing of the vessels. The feet are more generally affected first, but changes occur also in the blood vessels of the hands, and eventually the whole body.

Persistent coldness of the extremity is often the initial symptom. Numbness, tingling, and aching may be noticed. The feet may turn blue when lowered for long periods of time. Raynaud's phenomenon, intermittent claudication, and gangrene may also be present. Because of atrophy, there may be a decrease in the size of the leg. (279)

Jews have the highest incidence of Buerger's disease, but the disease is also common in the Orient. About 75 men are affected for each woman in the United States. (277) It has been observed at all ages, but is most frequent at 20 to 45. The incidence of Buerger's disease is decreasing in the United States.

Buerger's disease has alternating periods of activity and inactivity of the disease. It may necessitate the amputation of both lower extremities and sometimes the upper extremities if smoking is not controlled.

TREATMENT

1. Tobacco in any form must never be used as it produces vasoconstriction and probably favors extension of the disease. (277) Buerger's disease rarely occurs in non-smokers.

2. Increased coagulability (clotting) of the blood is thought to play a part in the disease. (278) Use a low-fat diet and maintain good hydration. Onions decrease clotting of the blood and may be of value.

3. Stay well clothed, paying particular attention to the extremities. The arms and legs should have as many layers of clothing as the trunk to assure balanced circulation. General chilling causes vasoconstriction and worsens symptoms. (278) Wear gloves and warm footwear in the winter.

4. Nervous tension sometimes worsens the pain. (278) Exercise neutralizes stress, and also improves circulation. Make it a part of every day.

5. The extremities should be protected from infection and trauma. Do not walk around barefooted. Wounds heal slowly and gangrene is more likely because of decreased blood flow. (278)

6. Exercise and activity levels of an individual have either a beneficial or harmful effect on his circulation. Exercise promotes blood flow in the arteries by alternate muscle contraction and relaxation, causing blood vessels to contract and dilate. Exercise is also one of the most important factors in the development of collateral circulation (the "sprouting" of new arterioles and capillaries from adjoining arteries to help supply blood to an area of blockage). Walking is one of the very best exercises for stimulating blood flow in the legs. (280)

Buerger's exercises are often prescribed for patients with vascular disorders:

A. Lying flat in bed, elevate the legs to above heart level for two minutes or until blanching occurs.

B. Sit on the edge of the bed, dangling legs over the edge. Exercise feet and ankles for three minutes or until feet become pink.

C. Lie flat for five minutes.

Repeat the exercises five times each, three times a day. (281) Gravity alternately empties and fills blood vessels and encourages development of collaterals. (282)

7. Chairs should be of a height that sharp knee flexion is avoided. Do not sit for long periods without getting up and walking. (280) The depth of the chair should allow an inch of space between the edge of the seat and the back of the knees. (280)

8. Women should not wear girdles and should avoid tight shoes.

9. A firm mattress should be used. A soft mattress may allow sufficient flexion of the trunk at the hips to hinder circulation to the legs. (280)

10. The patient should never cross his legs at the knee as this induces pressure on the popliteal blood vessels. He should periodically straighten the leg and rotate the foot at the ankle.

BURSITIS

Bursitis is inflammation of a bursa, a small fluid-filled sac located in joints to decrease friction between skin, tendons, ligaments, muscles, and bones. Trauma is the most common cause of bursitis, but infection, excessive use of the joint, allergies, and a number of diseases may induce bursitis.

Bursitis is slightly more common in women than in men because their shoulders slope more than men's placing increased pressure on the bursa. The shoulder is the joint most commonly affected by bursitis.

Because of overstimulation the synovial membrane produces excess fluid which causes distention of the bursa. It is this additional fluid and distention which causes the discomfort.

TREATMENT

1. Many cases of bursitis are due to overuse of the joint. Such

activities as painting, hanging wallpaper, and ironing for excessively long periods of time may induce it, and should be
avoided. Activities one is unaccustomed to should be done for
only short periods of time. Carrying a heavy handbag on a long
shopping tour can provoke a case of bursitis.

2. During the initial phase of bursitis ice applications are the
   treatment of choice. Apply an ice pack for 30 minutes every 2
   to 3 hours.

3. As pain decreases hot applications may be begun. Heat applied
   early in the course of the disease encourages accumulation of
   fluid in the bursa, making the pain more severe. Heat should be
   applied for 45 to 60 minutes, and followed with range of motion
   exercises at least once daily. The heat msut be as intense as the
   individual can tolerate.

4. Do not allow yourself to become chilled.

5. Exercises to increase blood circulation and prevent "freezing"
   of joints are often helpful. The following exercises are recommended for bursitis of the shoulder:

   A. Stand facing a wall at arm's length from it. Place both hands
      on the wall slightly above waist level, and "walk" hand-
      over-hand as far up the wall as you can reach. Repeat four
      to five times daily.

   B. Lean over at the waist until your chest is parallel to the
      floor. Make a motion with your trunk causing your relaxed
      arm and hand to swing in a circle. Try to increase the size
      of the circle from day to day. Make 15 to 20 complete
      circles.

   C. Raise the involved arm foreward and up, then backward and
      up, to the side and up. Raise the arm as high as possible each
      time. Repeat about five times each, daily.

   D. An overhead pulley with a five pound weight is often very
      useful. Pull the weight as high as possible. Begin with five
      pulls three times a day; gradually increase until you can do
      fifty pulls each time.

CELIAC DISEASE

Celiac disease is a disease of the small intestine characterized by
abnormalities in the intestinal lining due to a permanent intoler-

ance to gluten. Removal of gluten from the diet leads to full remission of the disease. (352) The word "celiac" comes from a Greek word which means "suffering in the bowels." (353)

Gluten is the germ protein of wheat, rye, barley, and oats, and perhaps buckwheat. (354) Gliaden is believed to be the toxic portion of the protein. The toxin causes the villi of the intestine to flatten and atrophy, causing malabsorption of nutrients and producing the signs and symptoms of the disease. (355) The same type of mucosal changes are seen in infantile cow's milk and soy protein intolerance, some types of gastroenteritis, giardiasis (a type of parasite) and some types of sprue. (356)

Onset of celiac disease is insidious and correlates with the introduction of gluten-containing cereals to the infant's diet. Because of the trend toward an earlier introduction of cereals into the diet most children's symptoms begin under one year of age. (352) Some patients, however, become symptomatic for the first time as teenagers or adults. (356)

Diarrhea is the most common presenting symptom. The stools are generally pale, loose, and have a very offensive odor. They may resemble oatmeal porridge. The child may have one large bulky stool per day, or may pass two or three. A few children may have constipation. Other symptoms of celiac disease are failure to thrive, vomiting, weight loss, loss of appetite, short stature, bloated abdomen, irritability, abdominal pain, frequent respiratory infection, sleep disturbances, edema, muscle wasting, pallor, muscle weakness, mouth ulceration, rectal prolapse, and skin infections. (352) Abdominal distention is felt to be due to excess gas from the fermentation of partly absorbed food. (358)

Elimination of gluten from the diet produces a dramatic clinical response, although total healing may take three months to one year. Weight often reaches the norm for the child's age within six months and height and bone age within one to two years.

As the lining heals, the patient will quickly replete nutritional deficiencies from the foods eaten, and only occasionally is it necessary to treat folate or iron deficiency. (356)

Some infants appear also to be intolerant of cow's milk protein, and may show symptoms of celiac disease from the milk before gluten is even introduced into the diet. (352) Elimination of cow's milk early in the course of treatment will often speed recovery.

TREATMENT

1. The earlier gluten is introduced the shorter the period before symptoms occur. (357) Avoid the introduction of wheat, rye, barley and oats as long as possible to allow the intestinal lining to mature. Rice, millet, and corn should be used in their place. All grains fed to babies (and adults for that matter) should be cooked for two to three hours if preparation is with boiling at 212 degrees F.

2. Breast feed the child to avoid the use of cow's milk.

3. Allisatin, an ingredient of garlic, is said to be useful in the treatment of celiac disease. (359)

4. Ripe bananas appear to be tolerated well (360) and may assist in the control of diarrhea.

5. There are differences of opinion regarding the use of buckwheat. Duncan Milne in his article entitled "Oats and Celiac Disease" points out that if the celiac is well, his diet is adequate; if he is not well, his diet, however official, is not adequate for him (361) and needs to be adjusted.

6. The patient must be strict in his gluten-free diet, carefully reading labels on commercially prepared foods for any form of gluten. Coffee and coffee substitutes may contain malt, wheat, rye, barley, or oats. Almost all commercial breads, bread mixes, crackers, muffins, cupcakes, rolls, RyKrisp, and pretzels contain gluten. Commercially prepared puddings, cakes, candies, cookies, ice cream, sherberts, etc., may contain gluten, and salad dressing is sometimes thickened or emulsified with products containing gluten. All breaded meats, luncheon meats, frankfurters, and canned chili must be avoided. Macaroni, noodles, spaghetti, and bread stuffings, many commercial soups and vegetables cooked with cream sauce thickened with flour, bottled meat sauces, condiments, flavoring syrups, gravies and sauces and cocoa mixes may contain gluten. (354) Breads and cereals made from rice, corn, millet, soybean, or potato starch may be used. Desserts should be homemade if used, but are best omitted from the diet. All fruits are acceptable, as are all frozen, fresh, or canned vegetables and vegetable juices.

CHIGGERS

Chiggers, also called red bugs, and "jiggers" are most common in the Southern United States, but are widely distributed from

Canada to Central Mexico. Chiggers are not insects, but belong to the class that includes scorpions, spiders, and mites.

Chiggers prefer grassy, weedy fields, but may be found in low, damp wooded areas, berry patches, orchards, lawns and parks. They usually have their greatest activity in June and July but any time from May to September can yield at least a few bites during an outing in the woods.

Once chiggers get on the body they tend to go to body creases and areas of the body where clothing fits tightly, such as armpits, knees, anklets, and under waistbands. About two hours are required for the chigger to find the place he prefers to bite. Then he inserts two pairs of grasping mouth pieces and a tiny forked claw into the skin through hair follicles or pores. It then injects a fluid which dissolves tissues, and produces welts on the skin. Itching generally begins three to six hours after the mites attach themselves, and lasts for about three days.

TREATMENT

1. After walking in the woods, or locations likely to harbor chiggers take a shower, scrubbing with a coarse washcloth or brush to remove any chiggers that have not yet become embedded.

2. After chiggers become embedded they need to be removed carefully. One may scratch them off with a fingernail or apply vaseline or castor oil.

3. Hot baths are generally very effective in controlling itching from chigger bites. A 20 minute bath as hot as can be tolerated will usually bring several hours of relief.

4. A charcoal poultice may be helpful.

5. A little water may be added to ground oatmeal to make a paste soothing to chigger bites. If the bites are widespread, one may add powdered oatmeal to the water used for a soaking bath. (523)

6. Banana is reported soothing to chigger bites. (524)

COLIC

Episodes of crying, fussing, irritability, and distended abdomen are symptoms of colic. The baby's face may be flushed, the feet may be cold, and often the hands are clenched. (77) Relief may come with a bowel movement or passage of gas. The symptoms generally begin after feeding and become worse late in the day. The infant may make sucking motions and appear to be searching for food. (78) Colic is common in the newborn, generally starting at two to four weeks of age, and usually ceases during the third or fourth month.

TREATMENT

1. Many authorities feel that colic is caused by an allergy. Babies who are bottle-fed may have clearing of colic by the removal of cow's milk from the diet.

2. Breast-fed babies may receive antigens through mother's milk. Eighteen mothers with 19 infants with colic were placed on a milk-free diet. Thirteen of the nineteen infants had prompt clearing of their colic. (79) Some physicians eliminate all dairy products (80) from the mother's diet.

3. Various other studies have indicated that cow's milk is the primary cause of colic, but such foods as chocolate, (79) banana, apple, orange, strawberry, coffee, (81) nuts, shellfish, (82) eggs, beef, veal, potato, wheat, navy beans, lamb, celery, (83) corn, tomato, onion, fish, legumes, citrus, and sweet potato (86) have been shown to produce allergic reactions. Test for these foods by eliminating them all from the diet, and add back one food every three to four days. If a food eaten by the mother produces colic in the infant it should be left off permanently.

4. Rocking the baby and singing to him may be helpful. (84) An old-fashioned cradle may be just the thing!

5. Automobile rides are soothing to some infants. (84)

6. One author reports that placing the colicky baby in an infant seat on top of a running clothes washer produces warmth and slight vibration which may sooth the infant. (82)

7. Feed the baby in a sitting position, and burp him after each ounce of fluid.

8. A pacifier may be helpful.

9. Formula should be given at body temperature. Do not over-heat it. (85)

10. Overfeeding (77) may produce discomfort.

11. Placing the infant on his stomach or right side is often helpful,

(87) particularly if a hot water bottle or heating pad is placed under his abdomen.

12. The mother of a breast-feeding infant should use a simple diet. The rates of colic increase in direct proportion to the diversity of the maternal diet. (88)

13. Inserting a vaseline-coated finger, thermometer tip, or glycerin suppository into the rectum may aid in the passage of flatus and prove beneficial. (78)

14. Several studies have demonstrated that drugs given during labor and delivery have an adverse effect on the infant and may play a role in the later development of colic. (89) This is one of many reasons to avoid drug use during this critical period of a child's life.

15. The mother of a colicky baby gave a supplement of Morton's Salt Substitute and lactobacillus acidophilus culture after having read the book, *Let's Have Healthy Children*. Four days later the infant became irritable and lethargic. He had a gagging episode and became cyanotic, apneic, and limp. He was admitted to the hospital where tests revealed a markedly elevated potassium level and bizarre EKG changes. (90)

16. Colic can be a perplexing and taxing ordeal for mothers. Often mothers benefit if they are able to leave the baby in the care of father or grandmother, and have opportunity to get away from the crying for a few hours.

17. Catnip or peppermint tea may prove soothing.

18. A one to two ounce warm water enema may assist in the passage of flatus or feces in the colicky baby. (91)

19. One-quarter of a bay leaf may be boiled in a cup of water for 15 minutes. Let it cool before giving it to the baby. If this does not produce relief increase the amount of leaf to half or three-quarters of a leaf, but do not exceed one leaf. (525)

20. Garlic oil may be helpful. (525)

21. Chamomile tea may be used to overcome colic spasms. (297)

22. Thyme is considered quite helpful in such gastric problems as colic. (298)

23. Anise seed tea (bruise the anise seed by rubbing them between two hard surfaces, such as the bottom of a drinking glass and the counter top) may be used in colic. (299)

24. Charcoal powder given by bottle is very helpful. One tablespoon of the powder stirred into four ounces of water is the
proper solution. One to two tablespoons of this mixture are
adequate.

CRADLE CAP

Cradle cap is the most common disorder of the scalp in infants.
(92) Symptoms vary from thin, whitish, flaky scales to thick, yellow,
greasy crusts. It may spread to involve the eyelids, external ear
canal, and nasolabial folds. (96) Approximately 50% of infants
develop it at one time or another. The exact cause of cradle cap is
unknown, but apparently several factors enter into it.

TREATMENT

1. Some studies suggest a strong allergic factor. Of a group of 187
   infants followed for ten years, 67% later developed an allergy.
   Allergy in the general population is rarely considered to be
   over 20%. (93)

2. Of the 187 infants studied, 135 of them developed cradle cap
   before they were three months old. The onset was nearly
   always three or four weeks after the introduction of a new
   food to the infant's diet. The cradle cap cleared with withdraw-
   al of the food. Foods most commonly observed to cause problems were milk, wheat, egg, and oranges, beans, and peas.
   Occasionally oatmeal was involved. (92, 93)

3. Inadequate scalp hygiene may play a major role in cradle cap.
   Parents are frequently afraid to shampoo the infant's hair lest
   they damage the fontanels (soft spots). However, the fontanel
   is like skin anywhere else on the body and will not tear or
   puncture with mild pressure.

4. Treatment is aimed at removing the crusts. Shampooing two to
   four times a week with a mild soap is helpful. Massage the
   scalp firmly enough to remove scales and flakes, but gently
   enough to avoid breaking the inflamed tissue beneath the
   scales. (95) If crusts are firmly adherent one may massage a
   vegetable oil into the scalp, allow it to remain for a few minutes, then shampoo it out. (96)

   An olive oil soap may be very helpful. Dissolve the soap in hot
   water until a thick lather is obtained. Rub the scalp with the
   lather, and rinse thoroughly with plain warm water. (94)

CROHN'S DISEASE

Crohn's disease, also called regional enteritis, is an inflammation of a part of the intestinal tract. It is quite similar to ulcerative colitis in many ways.

Crohn's disease, like ulcerative colitis, is more common in the United States and northern Europe, less frequent in central Europe and the Middle East, and infrequent in Africa and Asia. Ulcerative colitis occurs about twice as often as does Crohn's disease, but the incidence of Crohn's disease is rising while that of ulcerative colitis appears to be remaining stable. Somewhere between 5,000 and 10,000 new cases are diagnosed each year in the United States.

Blacks and Indians in the United States appear to be at low risk of developing Crohn's disease, while Jews seem particularly at risk. Jewish men have an incidence of Crohn's disease six times higher, and Jewish women three times higher, than non-Jews. Jews in Israel have a lower incidence than do Jews in the United States.

There appears to be a tendency for Crohn's disease to run in families; most often siblings are affected, less frequently parent and child. This may, however, suggest a common environmental factor more than heredity.

Crohn's disease is uncommon under the age of ten; the peak incidence occurs in the 10 to 20 year old group. (433)

The disease affects sections or regions of the intestinal tract, thus the name regional enteritis. The most commonly involved areas are the ascending colon, cecum and terminal ileum. There may be sections of normal mucosa between diseased areas. (434)

Symptoms are diarrhea and pain; but fever, weight loss, and abdominal masses may also be present. Abdominal pain may be made worse by eating and is improved by fasting, rest and local heat. Diarrhea is generally only four or five stools daily. Weight loss is common. There may be tenderness in the right lower quadrant and even a palpable mass in that region. There is often a history of aphthous ulcers.

TREATMENT

There is no known cure for Crohn's disease and treatment is directed toward relieving the symptoms.

1. Patients with Crohn's disease utilize fats poorly and do not tolerate high-fat diets well. A fat-free diet may greatly improve diarrhea.

2. Avoid foods known to be laxative.

3. Avoid gas-forming foods.

4. Condiments such as pepper, mustard, horseradish, and vinegar should be avoided. (435) Eliminate all food additives. These are all irritating to the colon.

5. Sugar and foods containing it should be avoided. A diet high in sugar may be related to the onset of Crohn's disease. One study revealed that patients with Crohn's disease ate considerably more sugar prior to the onset of the disease than did a control group of healthy people. (436) A group of Crohn's disease patients were placed on a high sugar diet and compared to a similar group of patients who were placed on a low sugar diet. On the low sugar diet four out of five patients improved, but nearly half of the patients in the high sugar group had to be taken off the diet because of deteriorating condition. (437)

6. Gluten may worsen symptoms of Crohn's disease. Four patients placed on a gluten-free diet for 12 days, then given gluten all suffered adverse effects within 9 days of the administration of the gluten. The adverse effects subsided within two to four weeks after the gluten was discontinued. (438) Gluten is found in wheat, oats, rye, barley and buckwheat. We have obtained striking results in some Crohn's disease patients with a gluten-free diet, but it must be rigidly adhered to. In sensitive patients, tiny amounts of gluten have been enough to cause exacerbation of symptoms.

7. Avoid stress, anxiety, and worry. Avoid competitive games and activities.

8. A fiber-rich, unrefined carbohydrate diet appears to have a beneficial effect on Crohn's disease. (439) Thirty-two patients placed on the diet had a total of 111 days of hospitalization during a four-and-one-half year observation period, while controls on the diet generally prescribed for Crohn's disease had a total of 533 hospital days. The increase in fiber intake should be gradual and food should be chewed thoroughly. Patients unable to chew well should blend or puree their food.

9. Fresh air and sunshine assist in the improvement of generalized immunity.

10. Crohn's disease patients have an unusually high incidence of allergic symptoms such as eczema and hay fever. (440) Eliminat-

ing the most common food allergens (Appendix A) for a one month trial period may prove beneficial.

11. Lactose intolerance is common. One study demonstrated that three out of five patients could not tolerate milk (441) and two of these had milk intolerance before the onset of Crohn's disease.

12. Charcoal may be helpful in control of diarrhea. Four to six tablets may be taken two to three times a day between meals. If the charcoal seems to irritate the colon one to three tablespoons of powdered charcoal may be stirred into a glass of water, the charcoal allowed to settle out, and the clear water drunk.

13. Patients with Crohn's disease were shown to have consumed prior to the onset of the disease considerably less raw fruits and vegetables than healthy controls. Raw foods may be protective. (436)

14. Avoid overeating as this may induce colon inflammation. (442)

15. Corticosteroids should be avoided. They initially may help the patient feel better, but they may actually precipitate septic complications. (443)

16. Antidiarrheal medications produce small bowel narrowing which can result in obstruction. There may be other unpleasant side-effects.

17. Surgery should be avoided except for treatment of life-threatening complications. Almost 50% of patients who undergo surgery report rapid progression of symptoms after surgery. (443)

CYSTITIS

Cystitis is an inflammation of the bladder. (97) The word "cystitis" is a combination of the words "cyst" (a hollow pouch, sac, or bladder), and "itis" (an inflammation). Symptoms are burning on urination, frequent need to urinate, and sometimes blood in the urine. Low back pain, cloudy urine, abdominal pain, chills, fever, nausea, vomiting, flank pain, and generalized "feeling bad" may also be present. (97) Cystitis is women's most frequent bacterial infection (98) but it is less common in men. Some 10 to 15% of women have recurrent bladder infections. Women's urethral and anal openings are much closer together than men's, and their urethras are considerably shorter, making it easier for bacteria to enter the bladder.

PREVENTION

1. Wash the perineal area with warm water after each bowel movement. Wipe from front to back to avoid transporting bacteria from the anus to the urethra.

2. Wear cotton underwear as cotton absorbs moisture more readily. Dampness and warmth encourage the growth of bacteria.

3. Shower instead of taking a tub bath. Such things as bubble bath, bath oils, excessive soap, and dishwashing liquid in the bath water are irritating to the urethra. Shower after swimming in a chlorine treated pool.

4. Use a mild brand of laundry soap. Rinse underwear several times as soap remains in fabrics. Boiling panties in plain water is often helpful.

5. Tampons may need to be avoided. They tend to be drying, may damage the skin on insertion, and contain chemicals in the cotton. Pads with plastic backing or chemical deodorants should be avoided. (99)

6. Dress to keep the extremities warm. Cold extremities force the blood back into the trunk, causing congestion. Anyone will remember having to pass urine after being chilled. The bladder and urethral nerve endings are stimulated by the cold. Shortly after passing the urine, the person feels the urge to void again, but this time has less urine to pass. The uric acid is concentrated in the bladder because of the lack of urine to dilute it, causing irritation. A warm shower to warm the body and drinking several glasses of water will assist in alleviating the situation.

7. Some cases of cystitis are on an allergic basis. (100) Eliminate the most common allergenic foods (Appendix A) as well as white flour, white sugar, sweets, cereals, onions and beans. Eggs are frequent offenders in allergic cystitis. If these foods are causing the problem, two weeks on the diet will bring some clearing of the problem. You may then begin adding these foods back to the diet. Barley, corn, and oats may often be used as they contain only small amounts of the protein which causes the sensitivity.

8. Some researchers recommend that a woman wash the perineal area before sexual activity and urinate afterward to assist in flushing out bacteria.

9. Birth control pills and spermaticides may cause cystitis.

10. Extra precaution should be taken just prior to and during menstruation. Menstrual products stimulate bacterial growth.

11. Maintain good hydration at all times. Hot climates are particularly dangerous as it is difficult to maintain proper hydration. Drink sufficient water to keep the urine pale. Urinate frequently to flush the system. One study showed that women who frequently suffer from bladder infections often have enlarged bladders from retaining their urine. As the bladder fills it compresses the blood vessels, decreasing blood supply to the area. (98) After voiding, the last few drops of urine should be forceably expelled to assist the bladder in its cleansing efforts. This procedure is a good measure of prevention.

TREATMENT

1. Avoid the use of antibiotics. They kill not only the bad bacteria, but the good as well. Yeast then has opportunity to overgrow, causing problems.

2. Drink large quantities of water—one-half pint every 20 minutes for three hours, then one cup every hour.

3. Camomile, goldenseal, buchu, mint, and parsley tea have all been used for cystitis. Do not add sweetener or milk!

4. Cranberry juice may be taken in place of meals, but for some this makes the burning worse.

5. Hot water bottles and heating pads may bring much relief. A hot water bottle placed in direct contact to the urethral and vaginal openings may be extremely helpful. If the skin around the urethra is warmer than the urine, the urine will feel cool rather than burning. (99)

6. A hot sitz bath (105 to 115 degrees F.) with a hot foot bath (110 to 117 degrees F.) for three to ten minutes is an old standby in the treatment of cystitis. Some people just soak in a tub of hot water.

7. A heat lamp may be used between other treatments.

8. Tea made with two or three crushed or blended bulbs of garlic may be drunk several times a day. (310)

DIVERTICULITIS AND DIVERTICULOSIS

Diverticulitis is an infection or inflammation of a diverticulum. Diverticula are saclike areas which balloon from the colon. Diverticulosis is a condition of multiple diverticula. About one in five patients with diverticulosis will develop diverticulitis. (377)

Diverticulitis and diverticulosis are not synonymous; diverticulitis requires inflammation and usually infection, while uncomplicated diverticulosis is essentially asymptomatic.

The primary symptoms of diverticulitis are pain, constipation, and fever. The pain may be localized in the left lower quadrant of the abdomen and may be constant. Some patients also have a brief period of diarrhea or a few loose bowel movements.

Diverticulitis is rare in people who eat a "primitive" diet high in fiber. As countries become industrialized, dietary habits change leading to prolonged bowel transit time, constipation, and increased pressure within the colon. These factors set the stage for the development of diverticular disease.

Pressure in a contracting colon segment generally decreases with increased bulk in the colon. Colonic pressure is normally about 5 mm. Hg, but if there is little waste material in the colon pressure may rise. This increased pressure is thought to produce ballooning of the mucous membrane, forming a diverticulum. (378)

At least 10% of Americans are felt to have diverticula. The condition is much more common in middle-aged and elderly persons than in the young. (379) Women tend to develop diverticular disease slightly more frequently than men, (384) which may reflect the greater likelihood of increased abdominal pressure from girdles and tight bands around the waist and abdomen.

TREATMENT

1. It is felt that diverticulitis may be prevented by avoiding constipation. The removal of indigestible fiber from foods with our refining processes may contribute to the development of the disease.

   A high-fiber diet can bring significant relief of symptoms in patients with diverticular disease, and the benefits increase with time. (380) Foods such as apples, peaches, bananas, pears, oranges, seedless grapes, seedless raisins, prunes, carrots, broccoli, lima beans, lettuce, turnips, bran cereals, whole grain breads, and miller's bran are all high in fiber. Foods with small hard seeds should be avoided as the seeds may become lodged in the diverticula. These include such foods as nuts, corn, popcorn, raw celery, tomatoes, cucumbers, grapes, figs, strawberries, raspberries, and breads with poppy, caraway and sesame seeds. (381) Chocolate should also be avoided. (384) Refer to the section on irritable bowel syndrome for a discussion on bran.

2. Dr. Thomas P. Almy, Professor of Medicine at Dartmouth Medical School told a symposium on nutrition and aging sponsored by the Institute of Human Nutrition that high intakes of refined carbohydrate, animal fat, and protein may also play a role in the development of diverticular disease. (382) Rats placed on high fat diets for 90 weeks all developed one or more colon diverticula. (383) Fat is felt to induce the secretion of hormones that alter muscle tone of the colon wall.

3. Use a low sugar diet.

4. Because constipation is considered so important in the development of diverticular disease, we recommend a diet low in dairy products. These are all constipating and contain no fiber. Twelve patients with diverticulitis with pain and frequent loose stools containing mucus and occasionally blood, were cured when they were taken off the raw milk they were consuming. (385) Another physician reported that two of his patients were cured on a milk-free diet. (386)

5. Exercise is important in the treatment of constipation, as are drinking plenty of water between meals and having a regular lifestyle with a set time for bowel movements. Try to have a bowel movement at the same time every day.

6. Use a heating pad to the abdomen for pain or spasm.

7. Baking soda, baking powder, spices, vinegar, and sugar may all be irritating to the colon. Their use should be avoided.

DYSMENORRHEA

Dysmenorrhea is painful menstruation. Symptoms include cramping pain in the lower abdomen, sometimes radiating into the groin, vulva and thighs. There may also be generalized discomfort, chills, headache, diarrhea, nausea and vomiting. Approximately 50% of women suffer from this problem which causes an estimated 140 million lost work hours each year. (109)

There are two types of dysmenorrhea: primary and secondary. The cause of primary dysmenorrhea is unknown. It generally does not occur until several years after menstruation begins. The pain generally begins a few hours before or with the onset of bleeding, and may last only a few hours or one to two days. It is generally worse on the first day and tapers off gradually. Menstrual flow is scanty during the maximal pain and flow increases as pain decreases. (101)

Several factors are known to aggravate primary dysmenorrhea: lack of exercise, poor posture, poor hygiene, nervousness, and such constitutional conditions as anemia, constipation, and habitually chilled feet.

Secondary dysmenorrhea may start two to three days before the onset of menses, with pain in the abdomen, small of the back, and radiating down the legs. It is not characterized by sharp cramps, but tends to be more constant. Symptoms continue throughout the entire period and sometimes even a short time afterward. Secondary dysmenorrhea is generally associated with some pelvic disease such as endometriosis, malposition of the uterus, inflammatory problems, tumors, etc. It is treated by removing the cause.

TREATMENT OF PRIMARY DYSMENORRHEA

1. A heating pad or hot water bottle to the abdomen often completely relieves the pain. A few hours of heat may enable the sufferer to resume normal activities.

2. Hot beverages such as herbal teas (alfalfa, red raspberry leaf, or chamomile) may be helpful. Avoid ordinary tea and coffee. Dr. Penny Budoff feels that the methylxanthines found in coffee, tea, colas and chocolate induce worsening of the premenstrual syndrome. (108) She reports that she and a group of patients who experimented with her had less breast tenderness after omitting methylxanthine-containing foods.

3. Regular exercise has been shown to relieve cramps in many women. In one group dysmenorrhea was one-third less frequent in those who exercised regularly. (109) A waist-bending exercise is the exercise of choice.

4. Some dysmenorrhea is felt to be due to poor posture. An exercise for improving posture is as follows: The patient stands about 18 inches from a wall with heels and toes together and the side to a wall. The elbow is put against the wall at shoulder height and the forearm and hand rested against the wall. Keeping the shoulders perpendicular to the wall and the knees straight, contract the abdominal and hip muscles and shift the hips toward the wall, attempting to touch the wall. The exercise should be done three times on each side three times a day, a total of nine stretchings per day. The study reported that mild cases reported relief after about one month of exercises, moderately severe cases after about two months, and severe cases after three or more months. (104)

5. Avoid constipation.

6. Overfatigue just prior to the period seems to make dysmenorrhea worse. Maintain a regular schedule of rising, exercise, and bedtime all month long.

7. Excessive pelvic congestion may induce dysmenorrhea. One physician who has studied dysmenorrhea says that women who have diaphragmatic (abdominal) breathing have no menstrual pain. Constriction of the breathing movements by tight clothing induces rib breathing, reducing the use of the abdominal muscles and diaphragm, and causing excessive pelvic congestion. She recommends the following exercise: The woman should remove all clothing and lie on her back on a flat surface. She should flex the knees and place the arms at the sides to assist in relaxation of the abdominal muscles. One hand is placed on the abdomen to assist in evaluating the amount of movement of the abdomen. The woman attempts to raise the hand as high as possible by lifting the abdominal wall and then to see how far she can lower the abdominal hand. The exercise should be repeated ten times morning and night in a well-ventilated room. Jerky movements should be avoided and a smooth respiration sought for. Initially this deep breathing may induce some dizziness, but with repetitions she will be able to complete the exercise. This exercise cured morning sickness in one of her patients.

8. The same physician suggested two hot tub baths a day at the onset of the period. The hot bathing draws blood from the over-congested uterus to the skin. (102)

9. Avoid the use of clothing which is constrictive. The extremities

should have as many layers of clothing as does the trunk to assure even distribution of blood throughout the body.

10. We have received reports that a four minute back massage an inch to the right of the lumbar ("small of the back") spine can bring relief for dysmenorrhea.

11. A hot sitz bath (105 to 115 degrees F.) with a hot foot bath (110 to 117 degrees F.) for three to ten minutes is often helpful. Some have occasionally used a cold sitz bath (55 to 75 degrees F.) for two to ten minutes with friction. (103)

12. Practice good posture at all times. Dr. L. J. Golub reported success with a twisting and bending exercise. The patient stands with the feet parallel and about 15 inches apart. The arms are outstretched to the side at shoulder height. Keeping the knees straight, the patient twists the trunk to the left, bending down and touching the floor with the right hand in front of the left foot. Return to starting position and repeat the exercise with the right foot. The first week the exercise should be done four times daily. During successive weeks the exercises should be increased by two each week until a total of ten repetitions per side are performed daily. Sometimes patients reported relief with the next period, but most people required several months before relief occurred. The author cautions that the exercises should not be started during a period as they may worsen the pain. (105)

13. A number of authorities recognize an allergic factor in dysmenorrhea. One study of 12 cases of dysmenorrhea reported that eight patients became free of all symptoms when the foods they were allergic to were eliminated from their diet. The other four patients received partial relief, and the author felt that he had not been successful in identifying all of their allergies. Wheat, eggs, milk, beef, chocolate, nuts, fish, beans, pepper, cauliflower and cabbage were the foods listed as the most common causes of dysmenorrhea. We suggest the elimination of all of the most common allergens (Appendix A) to test for allergy-induced dysmenorrhea. (106, 107)

14. Avoid overeating as this encourages abdominal congestion.

15. Sexual stimulation encourages abdominal congestion.

16. A low salt diet will assist in relieving bloating and water retention. (108) Even foods high in salt such as milk and other dairy

products, soy sauce, worcestershire sauce and monosodium glutamate should be avoided.

17. Lose weight if overweight. Obese women have a higher rate of dysmenorrhea than non-obese. (109)

18. Avoid smoking. The frequency of dysmenorrhea increases as the number of cigarettes smoked daily rises. (109) Nonsmokers had a 7.2% rate of dysmenorrhea; smokers had a 13.4% incidence.

19. Catnip tea each morning and evening during the period may be helpful. Chamomile is said to relieve menstrual spasms. Peppermint tea may ease the pain. (308)

GALLSTONES

Gallstones, called cholelithiasis by physicians, is the presence of stones in the gallbladder or its ducts. Gallstones are formed from bile, a brown digestive fluid produced by the liver. Between meals the bile is stored in the gallbladder where it is concentrated. When partially digested food passes from the stomach into the duodenum (the first part of the small intestine) it stimulates the gallbladder to send bile to assist in the digestion of fat.

The concentrated bile may become so saturated with cholesterol that some precipitates out and hardens into a crystallized form which is the beginning of a gallstone. These crystals irritate the gallbladder lining, making the gallbladder more susceptible to the bacteria which are often found in bile. This bacterial inflammation of the gallbladder is called cholecystitis. (316)

In the United States, cholelithiasis may occur in 10 to 20% of the population, and is more common in women than men. Pregnancy aggravates chronic cholelithiasis, perhaps because of increased pressure in the abdomen. Patients with diabetes, cancer of the gallbladder, cirrhosis and pancreatitis have an increased incidence of cholelithiasis. (317)

Symptoms of cholelithiasis are bloating, gas, and discomfort or indigestion after a heavy meal of rich, fatty food. Some patients have pain in the upper right quadrant of the abdomen, jaundice, chills or fever.

Often the patient has no symptoms, and does not even know he has gallstones until he sees his physician for another problem and they are accidently discovered. These are called "silent gallstones" so long as they do not produce symptoms. Physicians differ greatly in their opinion as to whether or not silent gallstones should be removed. In one group of 112 patients (318) the majority of them had no symptoms during a 10 to 20 year follow-up period. Three of the patients later died as a result of complications following elective cholecystectomy (removal of the gallbladder). Fewer than 20% of patients with silent gallstones may be expected to develop any type of significant complication within ten years of diagnosis, which certainly justifies watchful waiting. (319) The risk of pain decreases with the passage of time. (320)

TREATMENT

1. Dr. Mahantayya Math of Singapore reported that drinking water will help prevent gallstone formation. (321) He has observed that patients with gallstones consume little water. He feels that drinking sufficient amounts of water at regular intervals during the day, and late at night just before bedtime dilutes the bile, making precipitation of the crystals out of the bile less likely.

   Drinking 500 ml. (about one pint) of tap water induces emptying of the gallbladder 10 to 20 minutes later, which would decrease the amount of time the bile remains in the gallbladder.

2. A 15 minute hot fomentation over the gallbladder area, followed by an ice rub, repeating the process for three sets of change reduces the swelling and inflammation and eases pain.

3. Dr. Viado Simko reported to the Sixth World Congress of Gastroenterology that lack of exercise should be considered an important factor in the production of cholesterol gallstones. (322) Both animal and human studies indicate that there is a greater output of cholesterol and bile acids with the bile with exercise, but these changes were not present on days exercise was not performed. It required only 30 minutes of mild exercise, such as bicycle riding.

4. Some drugs are known to increase the risk of gallstones. Both clofibrate and oral contraceptives containing estrogen increase the cholesterol saturation of bile. (323) Excessive intake of vitamin B may lead to gallstone formation. (324)

5. A diet low in vitamin C frequently induces gallstones in guinea pigs. (325)

6. The low-fat diets used by some Asiatic countries are felt to be the cause of the low incidence of gallbladder disease in these countries. (326) A high fat dietary intake produces increased cholesterol content of the bile.

7. A high fat diet induced gallstones in a group of rabbits studied by Dr. Robert F. Borgman of Clemson University, but when Dr. Borgman gave the rabbits a high-protein, high-fat diet the incidence of gallstones increased. (327)

8. Food allergy is felt by many to be a cause of gallbladder disease. A 1968 study revealed that 100% of a group of patients were free from symptoms while they were on a basic elimination diet. Adding eggs to the diet induced recurrence of symptoms in a whopping 83% of patients! Foods inducing symptoms in the order of their occurrence were egg, pork, onion, fowl, milk, coffee, orange, corn, beans, nuts, apples, tomato, peas, cabbage, spices, peanut, fish and rye. (328)

   Dr. J. C. Breneman, author of *Basics of Food Allergy* feels that ingestion of the allergy-causing substance creates edema of the bile ducts, impairing drainage of bile from the gallbladder. (329) The inadequately drained areas are prone to infection, which forms the point of origin for cholesterol precipitations and subsequent stone formation.

   Patients with postcholecystectomy syndrome showed more favorable response to this form of therapy than to any other.

   Dr. Breneman points out that both gallstones and food allergies tend to run in families, and that migraine attacks are often associated with cholelithiasis. He feels that egg allergy is often the cause of both problems.

9. An increase of dietary fiber in the diet may make gallstone formation less likely. Bran decreases the colonic transit time, allowing colonic bacteria less time to act on bile salts. Bran may also prevent physical contact between the bile salts and bacteria. This produces an increase in the amount of cholesterol and bile acids excreted. (330, 331)

10. Refined carbohydrates and overnutrition are crucial factors in the development of gallstones. When fiber is removed from food it becomes less bulky, less chewy, and sweeter, rendering the food less satisfying, encouraging overeating. (333) An increased intake of calories, irrespective of their dietary composition may be one of the causes of gallstones. (332) All urban-

ized countries in which the diets are high in calories and fats have increased rates of cholelithiasis. (334)

11. Overweight people have an increased risk of developing gall-stones. Weight control by diet and physical exercise could substantially lower the incidence of cholelithiasis.

12. Animal protein intake is apparently associated with gallstone formation, while vegetable protein may actually cause some dissolution of gallstones. (335) A group of hamsters at Wistar Institute in Philadelphia were fed either soy protein or casein, an animal protein from dairy products. Fifty-eight percent of the animals given the casein developed gallstones, while only fourteen percent of the animals given soy protein had stones. We recommend a diet free from dairy products for persons likely to develop gallstones.

13. Two recent studies suggest that removal of the gallbladder may increase the risk of colon cancer. Cholecystectomy apparently almost doubled the risk of cancer of the right colon according to a University of Pittsburg study. The researchers feel that the higher concentrations of certain bile acids which reach the colon may induce cancer. These bile acids and their by-products induce cancer or serve as co-carcinogens in laboratory animals. (543, 542)

14. Chenodiol (chenodeoxycholic acid) has recently been introduced in the treatment of cholesterol gallstones. Reports are now coming in that many patients using this drug show elevated levels of cholesterol and low density lipoproteins which are associated with increased coronary heart disease risk. (528)

GAS

Gas, or flatulence, is the excessive collection of gas in the stomach or intestine. Belching may expel gas in the stomach, while intestinal gas is passed by the rectum.

Stomach gas is generally air swallowed by eating rapidly, gulping beverages, or using carbonated beverages. Its composition is generally similar to atmospheric air — 78% nitrogen and 21% oxygen.

Intestinal gas is generally produced by fermentation of starches and putrefaction of proteins. If an excessive amount of undigested food reaches the colon, the colon bacteria produce gas.

The gastrointestinal tract normally contains about three ounces of gas. Fermentation may increase the amount to as much as a quart, inducing symptoms of abdominal distention. About 90% of the gases formed in the intestine come from the breakdown of sugars, starches and cellulose (carbohydrates) and the remainder from protein. Methane is produced by one-third of the adult population as a familial trait, through bacterial action. It is not dependent on exogenous foodstuffs. Carbon dioxide and hydrogen are the main gases found with the fermentation of sugars and starches.

TREATMENT

1. Learn to eat slowly with the mouth closed. Don't talk while chewing your food. Saliva should be well-mixed with all foods as it contains substances which begin the digestion of food.

2. Mild exercise such as a leisurely stroll after meals mildly stimulates intestinal peristalsis. Lying down after meals, or sitting in an easy chair impedes peristalsis, giving greater opportunity for fermentation and putrefaction to occur. Lying down after meals may also interfere with the normal eructation of stomach gas. (174)

3. Activated charcoal adsorbs gas. North American Indians are known to have used charcoal for gas pains. (169) Thirty volunteers were fed bland meals, gassy meals, and gassy meals with activated charcoal capsules. They were asked to record their episodes of gas with each of the experimental meals. Volunteers reported that the gassy meals produced six or seven times as much gas as the bland meal or the gassy meal with charcoal. (179)

4. Laxatives may worsen gas by rushing undigested food particles through the intestine and into the colon.

5. Avoid tight-fitting clothes, especially girdles and belts. Men who wear suspenders have less indigestion. (168) Compression of the abdomen aggravates the situation. (178)

6. A sedentary job and/or lack of exercise induce sluggishness and decrease abdominal blood flow, causing defective absorption of gases. Have a regular schedule of out-of-doors exercise daily. (170)

7. People who sigh often swallow air. Sighing decreases intrathoracic pressure, and may tend to suck air into the esophagus. (177) Learn to be conscious of such activities.

8. Avoid the excessive use of hot beverages. People consuming hot drinks have a tendency to draw in air to cool the liquid.

9. Avoid the use of carbonated drinks, beer, champagne, and foods with air whipped into them (sponge cakes, milkshakes, etc.).

10. Avoid drinking from water fountains. To drink slowly and continuously from a glass discourages swallowing air as one drinks. When drinking from a cup, keep the cup tilted so that the upper lip is covered by fluid. Avoid drinking from straws or small-mouthed bottles. (178)

11. Meals should be eaten in a peaceful atmosphere, and in a leisurely manner. Eating hurriedly causes more gas to be swallowed with the food, and allows chunks of food to enter the stomach, where they cannot be properly digested. Exhale after chewing, and before swallowing.

12. Avoid chewing gum and smoking as these increase the amount of saliva in the mouth, causing one to swallow more frequently. Air is swallowed with the saliva.

13. Do not postpone bowel movements. Gas is normally passed during bowel movements, and if allowed to accumulate it will cause bloating and gas pain. (171)

14. Avoid foods known to cause gas. Milk is undoubtedly the number one offender in this area. One patient suspected that milk was causing his gas and drank nothing but milk for two days. He counted 141 episodes of flatulence. After eliminating all dairy products from his diet, his flatulence dropped to 25 episodes per day, a considerable improvement. (173)

15. Foods such as beans, navy beans, soy beans, lima beans, broccoli, cauliflower, peas, Brussel sprouts, kohlrabi, radishes, cumbers, celery, (178) corn, apples, raisins, bananas, prune juice, grape juice, and apple juice (174) have all been shown to produce gas. Onions and cabbage contain flavones which act to inhibit intestinal motility. Legumes, some fruits, and whole grains are also gas-forming in some individuals. (174) The oligosaccharides raffinose and stachyose which are found in beans are responsible for gas production. They are composed of several sugars linked by bonds that cannot be split by small intestinal enzymes.

16. A low fat diet may be helpful as it may reduce duodenal production of carbon dioxide. (175)

17. Avoid repetitive belching as belching almost always causes more air to be swallowed than is expelled.

18. Patients who tend to swallow air when they are under stress may place an object such as a pencil between the teeth to keep the mouth open.

19. Wheat ingestion may result in hydrogen production in normal subjects. Eliminating wheat may lower the quantity of carbohydrate reaching the colon. (180) Not all people will be troubled by wheat, but a wheat-free diet deserves a trial in difficult cases. White bread has been shown to be gas-producing. Use only whole grains.

20. Artificial sweeteners such as sorbitol and xylitol may produce gas in some individuals. (181)

21. Garlic relieved gas in the vast majority of cases in one study. Garlic apparently has a sedative action on the stomach and intestine. (182, 183)

22. Avoid overeating and thus overtaxing the digestive system. Eat meals on a regular schedule and do not eat between meals to allow the digestive system an opportunity to rest.

23. Drinking with meals dilutes the digestive juices, making them less effective. Learn to take meals without beverages and avoid much liquid food.

24. Many problems with grains and legumes may be because of inadequate cooking. Longer cooking increases the breakdown of starch particles, making digestion easier.

25. "There is no convincing evidence that simethicone, alone or in combination, is effective in the treatment of flatulence associated with functional disorders of the gastrointestinal tract." (184)

26. Keep well hydrated. A dry mouth encourages swallowing.

27. Anise tea is excellent for gas, particularly in children. (304) Spearmint tea may be used for flatulence. (305) Thyme tea has also been recommended. (306)

28. Treatment of acute gas pain:

    A. Pressure applied to the abdomen is often helpful in relieving gas pains. Lying on the stomach on a pillow is a common remedy.

    B. A heating pad on the abdomen provides relief for most people.

C. Rocking back and forth in the knee-chest position (kneel on a firm surface, place chest down on the floor, so that the head is lower than the hips) is often helpful. (176)

GOUT

Gout is a type of arthritis characterized by abnormal purine metabolism. Uric acid is the end-product of the breakdown of purine compounds. Gout most often affects the big toe, but may affect the ankles, knees, elbows, hands, and wrists.

The initial attack typically comes on suddenly in the middle of the night. There is severe, persistent pain in the affected joint. The joint becomes swollen and very tender, and the skin over the joint becomes red or purplish. Motion of the joint, or pressure applied to it, greatly increases the pain. After the acute phase, when the pain and swelling subside, the skin over the joint tends to itch and peel. Fever, loss of appetite, gastrointestinal problems, and decreased urine output are all common during acute attacks.

Gout seems to be increasing in incidence. It is much more common in males than in females; only about 5% of cases are in females. (216) Most males do not develop gout until after 35 years of age; peak age of onset is 45 years. Females with gout are usually postmenopausal. Gout tends to run in families. The mechanism may be that of a familial or genetic inability to excrete uric acid efficiently, coupled with a high dietary intake of purines.

Elevated levels of uric acid result in deposits of crystals of uric acid in the tissues, around joints, and in the skin and kidney tissues. These solid masses of urates are called tophi, and cause the inflammation, degeneration of cartilage, and overgrowth of fibrous or bony tissue characteristic of gout.

TREATMENT

1. Weight control is extremely important in the control of gout. Many people who have their first attack in middle life are overweight. Blood urate increases as weight goes up. (217) A person with gout should be 10 to 15% below his calculated normal weight. (218) Weight reduction must be done gradually as sudden weight reduction may induce acute gout attacks. (216) Fasting, even for a short period, markedly increases the plasma urate (a salt of uric acid); (217) do not fast with gout.

2. A high fluid intake has proved helpful in the treatment of gout. (218) The increased fluids help eliminate uric acid and slow kidney damage. Two quarts of water a day are recommended between acute attacks. Kidney stones (urolithiasis) are particularly common in patients with gout. About two-thirds of the uric acid disposed of each day is excreted by the kidney; the remaining one-third is broken down in the gut.

   About 20% of patients with gout develop kidney stones; the incidence of stones increases as the level of uric acid increases. The stones are pure uric acid in 84% of gouty patients; uric acid and calcium oxalate in 4%, and calcium oxalate or phosphate in 12%.

3. A diet high in unrefined carbohydrates and low in protein and fat may be helpful. A high carbohydrate diet tends to increase uric acid excretion, while a high fat diet not only decreases excretion, but may bring on a gouty attack. This occurs regardless of the saturation of the fat. (217) In Japan, gout incidence has increased as has protein intake. (216) Animal protein seems particularly harmful. Lord Horatio Nelson relieved his gout with a vegetarian diet. (219)

4. Uric acid is the end-product of the metabolism of purine compounds. A low purine diet produces a fall in plasma urate and has for many years been an essential part of the treatment routine for gout. Use a diet low in purines:

   Foods High In Purines: Liver, kidneys, brains, heart, sweetbreads, mussels, anchovies, sardines, meat extract, consomme, gravies, fish roes, herring.

   Foods of Moderate Purine Content: Fish except as noted above, other seafoods, meat, fowl, yeast, lentils, whole-grain cereals, beans, peas, asparagus, cauliflower, mushrooms, spinach, oatmeal.

   Foods Containing Negligible Amounts of Purines: Vegetables, fruits, milk, cheese, eggs, refined cereals, cereal products. (218)

5. Charcoal may be helpful in the treatment of gout. Charcoal compresses may be applied to the affected joint. Charcoal may also be taken by mouth and can lower the serum uric acid levels. Twelve to sixteen tablets should be taken daily.

6. Hot fomentations for 15 minutes every three hours may relieve

pain. Some people have better pain relief with cold applications. Use whichever is most effective for you.

7. During acute attacks keep the affected joint elevated and at rest so far as possible. Most patients are unable to bear even the weight of bed clothes on joints.

8. Any alcoholic beverage is contraindicated in gout. Alcohol not only increases urate production but also inhibits renal excretion of urate. (216) A group of patients given a purine-rich meal had an increase in serum urate levels of from 1.3 to 3.3 mg/deciliter. When the same meal was given with an alcoholic beverage, the increase ranged from 2 to 6.1 mg/dl. (220)

9. Colchicine is the usual gout medication. Side-effects of colchicine are nausea, vomiting, cramping, diarrhea, hair loss, suppression of bone marrow activity causing anemia, decreased leukocytes, decreased platelets and liver damage. (216) Most patients can be handled well without using pharmacologic agents.

10. Serum uric acid is consistently elevated by several drugs. The Framingham study showed that 50% of new cases of gout were diagnosed while the patients were receiving thiazides (a diuretic) or ethacrynic acid, a potent diuretic. (221) Penicillin, thiamine chloride, vitamin B-12, insulin, folic acid, sulfa drugs, ergotamine tartrate, as well as mercurial and thiazide diuretics have been implicated as precipitating factors in gout. Avoid the use of any drug. Obviously the extent of the problem has not been clearly defined.

11. Avoid the excessive use of yeast as it increases urinary uric acid excretion. (222) Food yeasts used for flavoring agents as well as bakers yeast will increase the uric acid level in the blood.

12. A considerable amount of uric acid is eliminated through the skin with mud packs. (223) At times the percentage of uric acid in the sweat reached a value equal to or exceeding that of the blood. Apparently the skin can extract uric acid from the blood.

13. A daily paraffin bath may be quite helpful in gout. Use a double boiler or crockpot large enough to accommodate the afflicted joint. Fill it about two-thirds full with paraffin, adding one-half to one pint of mineral oil per five pounds of paraffin.

The paraffin will melt as it is heated. With the temperature in the 125 to 135 degree range quickly dip the afflicted joint in the paraffin, withdrawing it immediately. Repeat the dipping several times, allowing the paraffin to cool and harden a bit between each dipping. When a thick coating of paraffin has been obtained dip the joint in the paraffin and keep it there for 30 minutes. The paraffin may then be peeled off and returned to the cooker.

14. There have been several reports in scientific literature of the use of cherries in gout. A group of 12 gout patients were given one-half pound of fresh or canned cherries daily. The uric acid level of the blood decreased, and no attacks of gouty arthritis occurred. Sour, black, Royal Anne or Black Bing cherries were used. One patient tired of eating cherries and began drinking the juice drained off cans of water-packed cherries apparently with equal success. (224) We have received reports of success with one tablespoon of cherry concentrate daily. If canned cherries are used, select water-packed varieties. Most brands are high in sugar and other additives.

15. There are some reports suggesting that gout may have an allergic component. (225) One case of a syndrome resembling gout has been reported in an individual drinking large amounts of milk. (226) When milk was removed from his diet the symptoms disappeared. Three cases of gout were linked to excessive tomato consumption in a 1977 medical report. One lady practically living on tomatoes and cucumbers developed gout for the first time.

16. Overeating may induce gout. (228) During World Wars I and II gout was uncommon in Europe, (216) and was exceedingly rare in Germany at the close of World War II. (229) It seems to disappear during times of decreased food supply.

17. Direct injury to a joint may bring on an acute attack. Avoid trauma to any joint known to be involved in a gouty process. (228)

18. A compress of comfrey root or leaves blended with water may relieve the pain of gout. (296) Spread generously on a square of paper towel or cotton cloth, large enough to extend outward well onto unaffected skin. Apply to painful areas overnight or for two or more hours.

HAY FEVER

Hay fever is also called allergic rhinitis. It generally occurs in the spring or fall, but people with allergies to such things as dust, feathers, or animal danders may have year around symptoms called perennial allergic rhinitis. Although hay fever is generally recognized as primarily due to inhalants, food allergies may play a significant role in the overall picture. Reduction of as many allergenic substances as possible is worthwhile. (478)

Symptoms of hay fever are runny nose, sneezing, and itching of eyes, ears, nose, and palate. There may be swelling of the nasal mucous membranes, cough, wheezing, difficulty breathing, and headache. Dry, windy days, riding in an open car, and working in the garden often increase symptoms. Morning and evening hours are the most uncomfortable; there may be slight improvement midday.

Ragweed and grass pollen are the most common causes of hay fever in the United States.

TREATMENT

1. Ninety percent of infants with hay fever showed improvement on a hypo-allergenic diet. (479) Milk, chocolate, eggs, corn, and citrus were the most common causes. Inhalants causing symptoms were house dust, mold, and pollen.

2. Cover mattress and pillows with plastic. Avoid wool bedding and furniture stuffed with horsehair.

3. Do not allow animals in the house.

4. Cold applications were effective in relieving one man's hay fever. Cold cloths wrung from ice water were applied to his forehead. As soon as they began to warm up they were renewed. Relief was obtained in about 45 minutes, but the treatment continued for three hours, then intermittently for six hours. The patient had no further attacks that season. The next year he had another attack and applied cold compresses for about four hours. In 24 hours he was completely relieved. (480)

5. Exercise will decrease nasal stuffiness. When the body is at rest blood vessels tend to relax. Three minutes of vigorous exercise has been shown sufficient to reverse this congestion. (481)

6. A hot foot bath is very helpful to relieve nasal congestion.

7. Hay fever victims should guard against chilling as it constricts

the blood vessels of the skin, driving the blood into other parts of the body, including the nasal cavities. The resultant swelling worsens symptoms. (482)

8. Chewing beeswax and the taking of bee pollen or horseradish have been recommended. We have not tried these methods extensively. Results to date have been minimal.

HICCUPS

Hiccups are intermittent spasms of the diaphragm. The noise results from the vibration of the closed vocal cords as the air rushes into the lungs. (117) Irritation of the phrenic nerve causes hiccups. Episodes of hiccups that last over a long period of time may be irritating to the patient, disrupting sleep and food intake.

Almost all hiccups are one-sided — only one side of the diaphragm contracts. (126)

The most common cause of hiccups is overeating or excessive drinking which causes the stomach to push or irritate the diaphragm. (126)

TREATMENT

1. A drink of water is often helpful. If that does not stop them, gargle with plain water.

2. Lying on the left side for 5 to 10 minutes may stop hiccups. (118)

3. Pressure with the flat of the hand applied to the pit of the stomach, below the breast bone has been used successfully. (119)

4. Although we do not know why, applying pressure to the eyeballs through the closed lids stops hiccups. (120) This maneuver is not recommended, since damage to the eyes could conceivably occur.

5. Another physician reports clearing a stubborn case of hiccups by standing behind a patient sitting on a chair. The physician grasped the neck gently with his fingers, and with his thumbs slowly massaged down each side of the spinous processes. This maneuver produced relief in a minute or two. (121)

6. Old standbys are rebreathing into a paper bag, and startling the victim.

7. Another maneuver to stop hiccups requires that the patient sit upright in a chair and hold his breath. He then extends his head as far as possible for 10 to 15 seconds, or as long as he can hold his breath. This maneuver apparently holds the diaphragm in a relatively fixed position. Sometimes it must be repeated several times before the hiccups cease. (122)

8. Catnip tea may be helpful. (123)

9. If a drink of water or catnip tea isn't successful perhaps a more complicated version of drinking water will be. Fill a glass with water and place in it a metal object such as a spoon. While slowly drinking the water, hold the upper part of the metal handle (with the lower part still in the water) against the temple. The author says he has used this successfully in hundreds of cases of hiccups. (124)

10. Changing the position of the uvula is often an effective treatment for hiccups. The uvula is the small finger-like projection in the throat that hangs down from the soft palate. The patient can look in a mirror, exhale, and touch the uvula with the handle of a fork or spoon. A cold utensil may be more effective, but is not necessary. After the treatment the patient should sit quietly for a few minutes with the head forward and the arms crossed over the chest, breathing shallowly to prevent recurrence of the spasms. (125)

11. A sneeze has occasionally stopped hiccups. The sudden inspiration or expiration overpowers the stimulus to hiccups and breaks the cycle to allow normal respiration to occur. (126)

12. A foot massage is sometimes helpful.

13. Bending at the waist to touch the toes, and holding the position for about sixty seconds will often cure hiccups in both children and adults. (271)

14. Ice is often useful in the treatment of hiccups. Swallowing crushed ice may be sufficient. An ice bag applied to the pit of the stomach is sometimes helpful. (272)

15. Light fingertip pressure on each side of the neck for about a minute has been reported to stop hiccups. (272)

16. Deep breathing may help, (272) as will simply holding the breath. First hold it in as long as possible, then hold it out as long as possible. A buildup of carbon dioxide has a sedative effect on the phrenic nerve.

IMPETIGO CONTAGIOSA

Impetigo is a common skin disease of childhood, generally caused by a streptococcal bacterium. It is more common in the southern and southwestern states and may be almost epidemic-like during the summer months. Lower socioeconomic groups living in crowded conditions are more likely to be troubled with it. (313) Peak incidence is in the two to eight year old group.

Minor trauma such as insect bites, cuts, or abrasions allow entry of the streptococci. An area of redness develops, followed by blister-like swellings. The lesions, if not scratched, will break down in four to six days, and form a honey-colored crusted lesion which heals slowly. The skin under it may lose its color; the color loss may be visible for months.

The lesions itch intensely and scratching leads to increased skin injury and inoculation of the streptococci in adjacent skin areas.

The face and extremities are the most commonly involved body parts.

TREATMENT

1. Removal of the crusts brings about a more rapid cure. (314) Bathing in soapy water every four hours during the day is recommended. More severe cases may require the use of normal saline or hydrogen peroxide diluted to one-fourth strength with water. Apply warm compresses or soaks to firmly adherent crusts.

2. A starch poultice may be applied if the lesions are centralized.

3. If the scalp is involved it may be necessary to cut the hair to treat the area.

4. Keep the fingernails short and clean to prevent reinfection. Wash the hands frequently during the day.

5. Change pillowcases and bed sheets daily. Boil all linens used by the patient for 10 minutes to prevent spread to other small children.

6. Use disposable tissues for handkerchiefs.

7. Do not swim. (315)

8. Exposure to the air will encourage drying of the lesions, making them easier to remove. Sunlight has antibacterial properties and may be quite helpful.

9. Use a simple diet without oils and sugars to assist the body in fighting the infection.

10. Have a set of towels and washcloths for each infected person.

11. Charcoal compresses may be applied overnight and used in the daytime between other treatments.

12. Hot and cold compresses may be used after removal of the crusts. Use water at 110 to 115 degrees for the hot compresses (3 minutes) and ice water for the cold (30 seconds). Use five changes with each treatment.

13. Lymph glands often become involved in impetigo. If this occurs, use a series of hot baths to raise the body temperature. The child one to three years of age may be put in a 107 degree tub of water for three minutes; older children may remain in the tub one additional minute for each year of age over three. Be accurate with the time as overheating may be quite uncomfortable. Keep the head cool with the use of a fan or washcloths dipped in ice water.

14. Isolate the child from others if possible.

INFLUENZA

Influenza is an acute, highly contagious respiratory disease of viral origin. It may occur sporadically or in epidemics, occasionally pandemics (world-wide epidemics) occur.

Three types of influenza virus are known; A, B, and C. Influenza is most commonly caused by type A virus. About every 3 years there are acute epidemics, usually in the autumn or winter. Major pandemics occur about every ten years when a change occurs in the prevalent type of influenza A virus. Influenza B virus causes an epidemic about every five years, but is rarely associated with pandemics. Influenza C causes only mild sporadic respiratory disease. (508)

Influenza virus is basically airborne, and most commonly spread by droplets containing the virus. The infected droplets are spread by coughing, sneezing, kissing, and the use of drinking glasses, towels, etc., which have been contaminated.

Symptoms come on about 48 hours after exposure and include fever, headache with light sensitivity, aching behind the eyes, chills, weakness, muscular aches and pains particularly in the legs and back, loss of appetite, sore throat, cough, and sneezing. The shedding of viruses in nasal secretions is increased by the use of aspirin.

After two to three days the fever subsides and other acute symptoms rapidly resolve. Cough, weakness, and fatigue may persist for several days or even weeks.

TREATMENT

1. Antibiotics do not have any significant beneficial effect on infections with influenza virus (509) and should not be used.

2. Increase fluid intake. Drink at least 10 glasses of water a day to help keep secretions in the lungs thin.

3. For sore throat that sometimes accompanies flu, gargle for 10 minutes every 2 to 4 hours using hot water.

4. A humidifier or steam inhalations may be helpful if there is chest congestion or nasal stuffiness. A shop lamp with a 60 watt bulb held one to two inches from the nose is a great help.

5. Irritating the nasal cavities and gargling with warm salt water is claimed by some to prevent influenza. Some researchers believe irrigation diminishes the likelihood of the influenza virus lodging in the nose. (511) This research points up the importance of properly dressing to avoid the slightest chilling, while avoiding overdressing which might induce sweating. Viruses grow well in warm environments.

6. Hot fomentations to the chest may aid congestion. Refer to *HOME REMEDIES* for procedure.

7. Hot foot baths may assist in relieving headache and nasal congestion.

8. Prevent overfatigue and chilling. Use warm, close-fitting bed clothes, laundered daily during the acute phase.

9. Back rubs may be given as a comfort measure and to activate the immune system.

10. The room should have a good supply of fresh air at all times, but no draft on the patient should be permitted. A draft is identified by its causing the patient's skin to become cooler than the forehead, or by discomfort experienced by the patient. Actually compare the forehead temperature with that of the backs of the arms, ear lobes, ankles, etc.

11. Take an enema at the first symptom. The bowels should be kept open, as respiratory viruses are shed partially through the gastrointestinal tract.

12. Do not smoke. Influenza incidence in one study was 21% lower in non-smokers (510) than in smokers who smoked 21 or more cigarettes per day.

13. Use a sugar-free, low fat diet.

14. A deep breathing exercise may be done every two hours or any time the patient thinks of it. Take a deep breath, hold for a slow count of 20, exhale through the nose, and hold breath out for a count of 10. Repeat 30 to 50 times. This procedure refreshes the blood to the tissues of the upper respiratory passages and carries away wastes and encourages healing.

INTERMITTENT CLAUDICATION

Intermittent claudication is a symptom of disease rather than a disease. It consists of cramping pain, weakness, and tension in a limb, usually the calves of the legs after muscular exercise. There is no pain at rest, and when the symptoms occur they are quickly relieved by rest. Intermittent claudication is often associated with such diseases as arteriosclerosis, thromboangiitis obliterans (Buerger's disease) and other occlusive arterial diseases of the limbs.

TREATMENT

1. Those who smoke more than 15 cigarettes daily have been shown to have a 9 times greater risk of developing intermittent claudication than non-smokers. People who smoke less than 15 cigarettes have a 6 times greater risk than non-smokers. (211)

2. A regular exercise program has been found very beneficial, particularly in those who were faithful in carrying out the exercises daily. The following exercises are recommended:

    A. Lie on your back on a firm surface. Rotate your ankles around in a circle.

    B. Tense the right leg muscles, lift the leg straight up, hold to a count of three, lower the leg, and repeat with the left leg.

    C. Still lying, rapidly bend and straighten alternate legs.

    D. Sit on a firm, straight-backed chair. Fold arms over chest, and slowly rise from the chair to a standing position, then sit down again.

E. Standing behind the chair, holding on to the back, stand up on tiptoes and slowly squat down to sit on heels. Return to standing position.

Exercises should be done at least once daily with ten repetitions of each exercise. Most patients feel better after six weeks of the exercises. (212)

3. In addition to the above exercises, the patient should take a daily walk. One group of patients was instructed to walk one hour morning and evening. They were to walk as far as they could go before pain developed, sit and rest until pain was relieved, then resume walking, repeating the process for an hour twice a day. At the end of six months over half of the patients were able to walk on level ground for as long as they wanted without pain. (213)

4. Some researchers feel that abnormally high blood viscosity can be the principal cause of poor blood flow. (214) To decrease viscosity, stay well-hydrated, and use a diet low in fats, sugars, and concentrated foods. Lowering the hematocrit to under 42 by blood donations was found to relieve pain in many patients with incipient gangrene of an extremity. Since stress increases blood viscosity, try to reduce stress as much as possible.

5. A series of hot baths were discovered to help most of a group of patients with early intermittent claudication. Each patient was immersed in a bath at 110 degrees F. The first bath may begin at 105 degrees F, and gradually raised. The water temperature was maintained at 110 degrees F until the patient's temperature reached 103 to 105 degrees F. Water temperature was then reduced to the mouth temperature of the patient and then maintained for an hour. A daily bath was given for 14 days. (215)

As with any prolonged heating treatment, the head should be kept cool by the use of cold compresses. Sponge the face and neck with a washcloth wrung from ice water, or place wrung out washcloths on the head. Change frequently as they warm up.

6. Elevated blood pressure levels (above 160 systolic or 90 diastolic) triple the risk of intermittent claudication. (211) Treat hypertension if present.

7. Diabetes may play a role in intermittent claudication. Eleven percent of a group of patients with intermittent claudication had diabetes, but only one percent of a control group. (211)

8. A total vegetarian diet, free of animal products, dietary cholesterol, and free fats and oils should be followed. Similar diets have been shown to induce regression of atherosclerotic lesions in both animals and men. Improvement in the large vessels involved in claudication is much slower than the dramatic results that are often seen in angina, however. (See section on Angina.)

IRRITABLE BOWEL SYNDROME

Irritable bowel syndrome is characterized by a change in bowel habits, abdominal pain, and the absence of detectable organic disease. Gas, nausea, lack of appetite, bad breath (336) heartburn, bloating, backache, weakness, faintness, and palpitations (337) may also be present. About 20% of people with irritable bowel syndrome have rectal bleeding. (338)

Irritable bowel syndrome seems to be a product of western civilization as it is unknown in countries where our refined diet is not consumed.

Irritable bowel syndrome affects from 50 to 75% of the population at some time during their lifetime. (339) It is more common in women. (340) Symptoms usually begin when patients are in their 20s or 30s; after age 50 the onset of irritable bowel syndrome is very rare. (341)

The bowel is generally structurally normal; the symptoms are due to an abnormality in function rather than anatomy. Instead of contracting in a coordinated way as in normal people, the colon muscles of people with irritable bowel syndrome contract in uneven spasms. This causes food to move through the gastrointestinal tract either too rapidly or too slowly. When it passes through too slowly too much water is absorbed, causing hard, dry stools. When it passes through too rapidly too little water is absorbed resulting in watery stools or diarrhea. (338)

There are three basic types of irritable bowel syndrome: (1) constipation, pain (2) painless diarrhea with mucus, and (3) alternating constipation and diarrhea. (346) Diarrhea frequently occurs immediately upon rising, and following breakfast. It may be accompanied by a feeling of urgency. The patient may be "constipated" for the remainder of the day. (345) Nighttime diarrhea is rare. (339) Some patients report pasty "pencil-like" stools rather than diarrhea. (337)

Basic electrical rhythm studies have demonstrated waves of either 3 or 6 cycles per minute. Irritable bowel syndrome patients have a significantly higher proportion of 3-cycle-per-minute waves under basal conditions (341) than do normal persons.

TREATMENT

1. Most patients have abdominal pain at times. This pain may be sharply aggravated by the intake of food or cold liquids, and may be relieved with an enema or the passage of gas. (342) A heating pad, hot water bottle, or hot fomentations applied to the abdomen will assist in pain relief. Moist heat may be more effective than dry heat as moist heat penetrates farther. One author recommends hot applications be applied for an hour, removed for an hour, and applied again for an hour throughout the day in severe cases. (343) Lukewarm tapwater enemas administered slowly may be very effective. (344) The pain is generally associated with periods of constipation. (346)

2. Because the passage of gas often produces relief of pain many patients feel they have excessive amounts of gas. Studies, however, show that the volume of gas is not increased in irritable bowel syndrome; rather the patient is unusually sensitive to normal volumes of gas. (340) The avoidance of gas-forming foods may decrease discomfort. (For a list of these foods see the section on Gas.) Efforts to reduce air-swallowing may be useful. Chew with the mouth closed. Keep well-hydrated to discourage trapping of air bubbles in thick, tenacious saliva. Chewing gum, carbonated beverages, smoking, sucking hard candies, etc. should be avoided.

3. Avoid xanthine-containing foods such as coffee, chocolate, tea, as well as spicy foods, some drugs, cold liquids and carbonated beverages etc., as these may induce diarrhea. (344, 346)

4. Milk may also induce diarrhea. As many as 70% of patients with irritable bowel syndrome have superimposed lactose-intolerance of some degree (347) and many of these patients may be "cured" by eliminating milk and milk-containing foods from the dietary. Even subjects who do not appear to be

lactase-deficient by conventional testing may not absorb a small fraction of lactose. Therefore a dairy-product-free diet should be tried in all patients.

5. Some physicians have suggested a relationship between food allergy and irritable bowel syndrome, and an elimination diet may be quite effective. It is felt that the offending foods act by direct irritation to the bowel.

   Patients should be instructed to keep a written record of foods eaten and note what foods are eaten within a 24-hour period prior to the onset of symptoms. This may point out a food or foods eaten before each attack. Sometimes foods may be tolerated in small quantities, but not in large amounts.

   Patients placed on the elimination diet (See Appendix A) may add one new food every three to four days, watching carefully for the onset of symptoms such as nausea, and gas. The most common offenders are milk, eggs, pork, wheat products, honey, sea foods, cabbage, cheese, chocolate and berries (343) and these foods should be the last added back into the dietary.

6. Eating meals on a regular schedule encourages the bowels to move regularly. Irritable bowel syndrome patients should be particularly careful to eat slowly, chewing the food well as this is necessary to stimulate the colon to move the residue along. (343) Avoid overeating which places an additional burden on the colon. Large meals are likely to be followed by a bowel movement. Put at least five hours from the end of one meal to the beginning of the next to allow the "interdigestive phase" to cleanse the bowel and encourage healing of the irritability. (See Appendix F.)

7. Stress plays a prominent role in the flaring up of irritable bowel syndrome. Regular, moderate, out-of-door exercise serves as a "nerve sedative" and relaxes the nervous system, a condition of great value to those suffering from irritable bowel syndrome. (343) Participation in an enjoyable form of vigorous physical exercise at least four or five times weekly is a way to defuse anxieties and stresses. (348) Exercise also restores the patient's confidence in his physical capacities. (342)

8. Cigarette smoking must be avoided; it irritates the bowel.

9. Avoid laxatives as these may induce colonic dysfunction. (343)

10. Massage over the abdomen may be helpful to induce healing and during periods of constipation. (343) Slow, light, continuous stroking is useful when abdominal muscles are weak and the colon is spastic. Occasionally deep pressure with kneading and rolling may be helpful.

11. "Drug therapy should be avoided if at all possible," (340) and we have always found ways to avoid drugs.

12. A diet high in fiber has been shown quite helpful in irritable bowel syndrome. Some researchers feel that an irritable bowel is one that is irritated by a refined, fiber depleted diet. (349) Patients in the study demonstrated greater relief of symptoms at three months than at six weeks, so the diet should be used persistently.

    Patients should be instructed to take only two teaspoonsful of bran three times daily for the first two weeks, and then they may gradually increase the amount taken until they can pass their stools without straining. It may take some patients two months to work up to this level. (350) Initially the patient may have increased levels of gas and distention but patients should persist in the program as these symptoms often disappear within three weeks of the start of the program.

    Thirty patients were instructed to take eight to ten rounded teaspoons of unprocessed bran within the same four to six hour period each day. Twenty-three of the patients reported that their stools increased in volume and their bowel habits became more regular. There was a marked decrease in cramps and abdominal distention. (351)

    Coarse bran has a more favorable effect than fine bran. (336)

13. Dr. T. L. Cleave who has done extensive research on the effects of a high fiber diet states that the refining of sugar is eight times greater than the refining of white flour, and feels that the elimination of refined sugar and all foods containing it is essential in irritable bowel syndrome. (350)

KIDNEY STONES

Kidney stones are also called renal calculi or urolithiasis. Stones may be formed anywhere in the urinary tract, but the kidney is the most common site. They vary in size from a grain of sand to an orange.

Kidney stones occur most frequently in the third to fifth decade, and are more common in men than in women. Approximately 200,000 people a year are hospitalized in the United States due to stones. (444)

A sharp, severe pain of sudden onset is the most common symptom of a kidney stone. There may be nausea, vomiting, blood in the urine, paleness and sweating.

Kidney stones are composed of one or more of the following substances: calcium oxalate, uric acid, struvite (magnesium ammonium phosphate) or cystine. Calcium oxalate stones are the most common type in the United States. (444)

Calcium oxalate stones may contain calcium phosphate. The milk-alkali syndrome and overdoses of vitamin D are known to cause calcium oxalate stones. Patients who take excessive alkali may produce calcium phosphate stones. A high purine diet (see gout) may induce uric acid stone formation. (445)

TREATMENT

Dietary Guidelines

1. A diet low in protein has been shown to be helpful to a group of patients who had recurrent uric acid stones. (446)

2. Milk may contribute to the formation of kidney stones. Studies at the University of Chicago showed that both lactose and calcium were involved in stone formation. (448)

3. Become a teetotaler. Alcohol consumption has been shown to injure the urinary system and to encourage kidney stones. (449)

4. Since a diet high in refined carbohydrates (sugar) (450) and possibly white flour products may increase the risk of calcium stone formation, use extremely sparingly or avoid entirely all concentrated sweeteners such as sugar, honey, syrup, and molasses. Even refined grains are suspected (white flour products, white rice, etc.)

5. Animal flesh increases urinary oxalate (451) and should be avoided. Proper vegetarian diets are recommended. The risk of stones in a population is related to the consumption of animal protein. (452)

6. A low fat diet should be taken. A 1981 study reported in the *British Journal of Urology* revealed that the percentage of calo-

ries provided by fat was higher in stone formers than in non-stone formers. (453)

7. Oxalate stone formers should avoid high oxalate foods such as tea, chocolate, cocoa, coffee, cola drinks, beer, citrus fruits, apples, grapes, cranberries, beans, rhubarb, beet greens, polk weed, chard, endive, and spinach, almonds, cashews, sweet potatoes, tomatoes, okra, figs, gooseberries, plums, currants, and raspberries. (484, 457)

8. Worcestershire sauce has a number of ingredients which are toxic to the kidneys and are felt to cause kidney stones. (456) Leave condiments alone.

9. Bran given to a group of 30 patients reduced urinary calcium excretion 20 to 25% in 22 of them. Researchers feel the reduction is sufficient to cut in half the risk of stone formation. The patients were given 24 grams of unprocessed bran in divided amounts with each meal. (458)

Avoid Supplements

10. Avoid vitamin C supplements. Ascorbic acid in large doses may increase the urinary excretion of oxalic acid, which may activate stone formation. (447)

11. Vitamin D supplements and vitamin D enriched foods stimulate parathyroid hormone production and should be avoided. (444)

Hydrotherapy

12. The simplest, safest, and most important therapy for kidney stones is a high fluid intake. (451) Patients should drink one glass of water every hour during the day and two glasses just before going to bed. (444) If they awaken during the night they should drink another glass. The increased urine volume decreases the concentration of solutes and prevents urinary stasis. Drink extra if you are perspiring heavily.

13. Buchu tea has a diuretic effect and may be taken as a part of the fluid intake.

General Measures

14. Lying down slows renal drainage and alters calcium metabolism. (454) Try to be physically active, with daily out-of-doors exercise. Bedridden patients are more likely to form stones.

15. Urine may be strained easily by placing two unfolded gauze

sponges in a funnel. The physician may have the stone ana-
lyzed to determine what type it is to assist in determining what
foods to avoid and general measures to pursue.

16. Analgesics such as aspirin have been shown to increase stone
    formation. (455) It is best to avoid all drugs as any are poten-
    tially injurious to the kidneys.

MASTITIS

Mastitis is an inflammation of the breast. It generally occurs
between the fifth day post-partum, to the second or third week,
and normally is limited to one breast. Symptoms include inflammation, redness, pain, fever, chills, headache, and malaise. Mastitis
should be treated promptly to prevent abscess development. If
treated within 12 to 18 hours of the first symptoms, abscesses are
generally avoided. (132)

Mothers nursing their first baby are particularly susceptible.
(127)

PREVENTION

1. Preventing mastitis is easier than treating it once it occurs.
   Mothers should be taught to wash their hands before handling
   their breasts.

2. If the infant is not permitted to nurse too long at one breast
   the possibility of fissures of the nipple is decreased. Some physicians limit feeding periods to five minutes on each breast for
   the first few days. (131) Bacteria enter the bloodstream more
   readily with fissures.

3. If the mother inserts a portion of the areola (the brown portion of the nipple) into the infant's mouth, his jaws will compress the milk pockets instead of merely the tip of the nipple,
   and prevent much soreness. (128) Rubbing the nipple a bit will
   encourage it to become firm and stand out so it is more readily
   grasped by the infant. Pinching the areola flattens the nipple to
   fit the infant's mouth better. At the end of feeding, to disen-
   gage the infant, place a finger inside the corner of the infant's
   mouth to allow air to enter the mouth and break the vacuum.
   After each nursing period it is very important that the nipples
   be washed with clear water to remove all saliva, as it contains
   an enzyme which will soften the skin. Water or alcohol applied

to the nipples will toughen the skin and assist in preventing sore nipples.

4. The nipples should be checked daily and if they are sore or cracked treatment should begin promptly. This is important. Do not wait until the condition is well developed to begin treatment.

5. Exposing the breasts to the air for 20 minutes at a time two or three times a day is helpful. (129) The nipples may also be exposed to an ordinary lamp with a 40-watt bulb for 15 to 20 minutes, held 1 to 2 inches away from the breasts.

6. Mothers should not use soap on the breasts as it is excessively drying and may lead to cracking.

7. Plastic liners in the bra should be removed as they hold in moisture. If troubled with breast leakage, the mother should use something absorbent such as a folded handkerchief to absorb the moisture, changing it frequently as it becomes damp. (130)

8. Changing nursing position for each feeding assures that different areas of the nipple are subjected to the stress from sucking.

9. Feeding the baby before the breasts become so enlarged that the infant has difficulty grasping the breast is recommended. Stasis of milk is an important factor in the development of mastitis. (133) The theory is that the milk-distended ducts provide an environment favorable for bacterial growth. (134) The over-distended breasts are difficult for the baby to grasp.

10. If the baby is fed before he is overly hungry, he will not suck the nipple too vigorously. Do not allow the infant to chew and macerate the nipple, opening the way for bacteria.

11. If the nipples become sore, an application of cold tea, which contains tannic acid, can promote healing. (130) Ordinary pekoe tea or a special tea from the health food store is satisfactory for this use. Moisten a folded facial tissue in the tea, lay it over the nipple for 20 minutes, dry and expose to air for 20 minutes. Rinse nipple before the next nursing.

TREATMENT

1. Alternate hot and cold compresses are often all the treatment required. Apply a hot compress for three minutes, then cold

for 30 seconds, with three changes. The treatment should be given two or three times a day.

2. Some women prefer a continuous cold application, such as an ice bag. Use a hot foot bath with the cold. (135)

3. Mothers should nurse the affected breast twice as often, but for shorter periods of time. (134) Try to keep the affected breast emptied.

4. The breasts should be well-supported by a bra. (133)

5. The mother should be careful to obtain plenty of rest during this period. Frequent rest periods during the day are recommended.

6. For many years physicians recommended that mothers with mastitis stop nursing their infants, but now it is known that to continue nursing is the best procedure. One study reported that mothers who continued nursing their babies recovered in an average of three days, and none of the infants were injured by the nursing. A control group of 30 women stopped nursing, and some of them had persistent infections for an average of two months. Half of them had to have drainage of one or more abscesses. (136)

7. Poultices of comfrey root or leaf may be used for sore nipples. (311)

MENIERE'S DISEASE

Meniere's disease accounts for about 5% of all dizziness, and 10 to 15% of all vertigo (a sensation that the world is moving around one). It generally occurs in adults and consists of recurring episodes of ringing in the ears (tinnitus) and hearing loss, and a feeling that the room is spinning. Patients often report a sensation of "fullness" in the ears. The vertigo may last hours or days, occur every week, or go ten years without a recurrence. Eighty to ninety percent of patients have hearing loss only on one side. (252) The disease may progress until the patient is completely deaf in the afflicted ear. (253)

The cause of Meniere's disease is unknown, but it may be related to a dysfunction of the autonomic nervous system which produces a constriction of the blood vessels which supply the inner ear. (253)

Meniere's disease most commonly occurs in women 50 to 60 years of age. The onset is sudden, and without warning. Sudden movement of the head during an attack may induce nausea and vomiting. There may be uncontrollable horizontal jerking of the eyeballs.

Patients often have a history of allergies, vasomotor rhinitis, and ear trouble. (256)

TREATMENT

1. Use an oil-free diet to improve blood circulation in the tiny capillaries.

2. Smoking induces vasospasm and vasoconstriction and should be eliminated.

3. Lying quietly on the affected side with eyes turned in the direction of the affected ear may assist in relieving the attack. (253)

4. Patients should be allowed to move at their own rate, and be protected from sudden moving and jarring as this aggravates vertigo.

5. Persons speaking to victims of Meniere's disease should stand directly in front of them so the patient does not have to turn his head.

6. The patient should not try to read and should be protected from bright lights.

7. Several studies have shown a relationship between Meniere's disease and diet. Dr. Roger Boles, of the Department of Otolaryngology of the School of Medicine at the University of California reports that almost 9 out of 10 Meniere's disease patients are greatly improved on a strict low-salt diet. (254) (See Appendix D for a low-salt diet.)

8. Diuretic teas such as watermelon seed, buchu, burdock, and cornsilk may be helpful. Asparagus shoots have a diuretic action. (300)

9. Some cases of Meniere's disease may be due to food allergies. Dr. Jack Clemis, an associate in otolaryngology at Northwestern University Medical School reports that allergies to milk, eggs, corn, wheat, and yeast are sometimes the cause of Meniere's. Eliminating these foods from the diet results in

clearing of Meniere's disease. (255) We suggest the exclusion of the most common food allergens (see Appendix A) for a month, then reintroducing one food at a time about a week apart. If symptoms recur, eliminate the food.

10. Dr. William A. Updegraft, director of the Department of Otolaryngology at Vassar Brothers Hospital, Poughkeepsie, New York, says that the most common cause of vertigo is a disorder of glucose metabolism. (257) He observed that variations from normal in glucose tolerance testing are very frequently accompanied by dizziness. When insulin levels are normal the patient seldom has tinnitus, vertigo, fullness in the ear, or fluctuant hearing loss.

Dr. T. S. Danowski, Professor of Medicine at the University of Pittsburg School of Medicine has developed a system involving a glucose tolerance sum. He tabulates the sum of fasting, one-half hour, one hour, and two hour blood sugar levels. If the sum is under 500 mg per 100 ml., there is no diabetes and vertigo is rare. A sum between 500 and 800 mg. per 100 ml., he calls a prediabetic or chemical diabetic state. Vertigo is common in this range. A total of over 800 mg. per 100 ml. indicates diabetes. A stable diabetic with little glucose fluctuation rarely has vertigo, but with wide swings in blood sugar levels dizziness is frequent. Dr. Danowski gives his patients a healthful diet and all but half a dozen patients in a three-and-a-half year study period have had no recurrence of dizziness. The use of the pancreas recovery program will assist in normalizing any blood sugar problems present. (See Appendix E.)

11. Daily exercise out-of-doors will assist in improving the circulation to the inner ear.

12. Stay well-hydrated to keep the blood from becoming excessively thick, hindering proper flow.

MIGRAINE

Migraine headaches occur in 10 to 20% of the population, and affect children as well as adults. (231) Pain is most common in the temple but may occur anywhere in the head, face, or neck. (230) A migraine attack is generally one-sided, but the pains may change to the opposite side, alternate sides, or occur on both sides of the head. (232) It is felt that 15 to 19% of men and 25 to 29% of women suffer a migraine attack sometime during their lifetime. (233) Probably half of all migraine sufferers do not consult a physician. (232) Numerous factors may induce headache, but six factors are felt to be the most common: food allergy, hypoglycemia, tension, depression, water retention, and menstruation. (234) Women often report a relationship between menstrual periods and migraine. Times of hormonal change as occur in menstruation, ovulation, menopause, etc., tend to worsen migraine. Discontinuing oral contraceptives may result in marked improvement in symptoms. Menopause may bring some relief, but many postmenopausal women have an increase in the frequency and intensity of the headaches. (232) Many women report that pregnancy improves migraine, and after the first trimester they are free of attacks.

Migraine has periods of remission and exacerbation; after decades of quiescence they may suddenly reappear. (232) Past middle age, attacks often seem to decrease in frequency and intensity.

Migraine sufferers often have prodromal symptoms before the onset of the actual migraine. These symptoms are such things as light sensitivity, bright spots and patterns before the eyes, mood changes such as euphoria, drowsiness, thirst, and hunger, insomnia and fluid retention. (235) The pain of migraine is severe, throbbing, and increases to maximum within an hour after onset. Nausea, vomiting, irritability, and light sensitivity are often associated with intense pain. If untreated most headaches will last 8 to 12 hours, but some may persist for 24 or more hours.

Migraine headaches are thought to be due to temporary changes in the blood vessels of the scalp and brain. It is believed that the prodromal visual symptoms are due to narrowing of the blood vessels, and the headache to their widening after the constriction.

A tendency to migraine may run in families; over 50% of the patients report that one or both of their parents suffered from migraines. (235)

TREATMENT

1. It is felt that over 25% of migraines are due to food sensitivities. (236) More than 2000 years ago, Hippocrates recognized a relationship between milk and headaches. (237) Since then there have been numerous studies confirming this. Other foods commonly associated with migraines are chocolate, cola drinks,

corn, pork, onion, garlic, (238) wheat, citrus, eggs, tea, coffee, beef, cane sugar, yeast, (239) cheese, alcoholic drinks, fried foods, seafood, (237) peas, and mushrooms. (239) Patients are usually allergic to more than one food group. (242) If you suspect that a specific food is causing your migraine, eliminate it from your diet for five days, then eat only that food for one meal. If you develop a migraine eliminate the food from the diet. (236)

If one is tired, anxious, or has missed the previous meal, a headache is more likely to occur if one eats a food he is sensitive to.

2. Tyramine, a breakdown product of the amino acid tyrosine, induces migraines in a significant number of selected migraine patients. Substances that have undergone bacterial decomposition have high levels of tyramine. The tyramine content of cheeses varies according to the aging time of the cheese. Avocados, raspberries, plums, orange, and banana all contain small amounts of tyramine. (237) Foods containing tyramine should not be used by migraine sufferers. It is felt that tyramine releases norephinephrine from the tissue stores in the brain, causing the blood vessels of the scalp and brain to constrict. The decreased blood supply induces the visual symptoms often seen before the onset of the pain. When the supply of norepinephrine is exhausted, the scalp vessels rebound from constriction by dilating, inducing severe head pain. (244)

3. Of a group of 500 migraine patients, 18% reported that fatty fried foods caused them to have migraines. (237) A fat free diet (see Appendix C) would probably be helpful to many. Do not reuse oil in frying.

4. Smoking may precipitate severe migraine headaches. (239) Even other people's cigarette smoking may induce headache.

5. Chocolate rates high as a cause of migraines. (240) Chocolate contains high levels of sugar which rob the body of B vitamins. Severe vitamin B deficiency is often observed in patients suffering from migraine. (241) Chocolate contains alkaloids which are toxic, and often contaminants of insect and rodent parts can cause migraine.

6. Refined carbohydrates should not be used. They are second-class foods, even for people without migraines.

7. Caffeine is known to cause migraine. Avoid coffee, tea, colas,

chocolate, and other caffeine-containing foods. Many medications including some commonly used in the treatment of migraine, contain caffeine! (238)

8. Food additives such as sodium nitrite, sodium glutamate, and tartrazine, (237) vinegar, and monosodium glutamate may induce headache.

9. Some migraine patients have increased headache frequency while taking antibiotics. It is felt that the antibiotics alter the intestinal flora, resulting in increased putrefaction. (237) Allergy shots may cause migraines. (238)

10. A high salt load induced migraine in 10 of 12 patients in a 1976 study. A handful of salted nuts or potato chips is sufficient to produce migraine in susceptible individuals, particularly if taken on an empty stomach. It may take six to twelve hours from the salt ingestion to the onset of the migraine. (243)

11. Odors and inhalants may trigger migraine. (245) Tobacco smoke is probably the most common of the odors, but perfumes, engine exhausts (particularly diesel), smog, paint, paint thinners, aerosols, frying odors, flowers, chlorine, ammonia and formaldehyde present in some permanent press fabrics are all known to induce migraine. House dust and molds are the most common of the inhalants, but pollen and animal danders may also be involved.

12. Chills may induce migraine. (238)

13. Emotional stress and resentment are said to precipitate migraine attacks. (235)

14. Rest in a darkened room with an ice cap to the head is helpful. (235) One physician reported success in treating his migraine with ice to his forehead. He states that within three minutes there is aggravation of the pain, and nausea, but within a few seconds all symptoms disappear, except for a very mild headache. (246)

15. Six patients in a 1982 study were able to abort their migraine attacks by rebreathing into a paper bag for 10 to 20 minutes. (247)

16. The frequency of migraine attacks decreased 50% in a group of adults placed on a vigorous, regular exercise program. (248) The exercise may inhibit blood platelet aggregation or decrease sympathetic activity.

17. A hot foot bath may relieve migraines. When the feet and ankles are immersed in hot water, the blood vessels dilate, drawing blood from the congested tissues of the head. Keep the water as hot as can be tolerated by adding more hot water.

18. Dr. Augustus Rose of the Veteran Administration Wadsworth Medical Center in Los Angeles has treated migraine by instructing his patients to take a hot shower, then a cold one. (249) The hot shower should include the head and be long enough to induce redness of the skin, and the cold must be long enough to induce shivering.

19. Exposure to sunlight triggered migraine in 30% of a group of 263 patients. (250) Most of the patients had to be out in the sun for at least one-half to one hour and the sun had to be bright. Staying in the shade on sunny days did not induce migraine. Wearing dark glasses was sometimes helpful.

20. Maintain a regular schedule. Extra sleep, too little sleep, or missing meals, may trigger attacks. (251) Napping or sleeping late should be avoided. Meals on a regular schedule enable the body to adjust its circadian rhythm of digestive juices, decreasing intestinal fermentation and putrefaction.

21. An enema may stop migraine in the early stages. (274)

22. Wrapping a tight bandage around the head may compress the swollen blood vessels and abort a migraine in the early stages. (274)

23. Throbbing head pain may sometimes be relieved by light pressure on the arteries of the neck. (274) Locate the pulse on each side of your neck and with your fingertips apply light pressure for a few seconds at a time. (274)

MUSCLE CRAMPS

Muscle cramps may occur in any muscle in the body, but they are most common in the legs and feet. Fifty percent of people between the ages of 15 and 80 years of age will have pain, cramps, or abnormal sensations of the legs at some time during their lives. (137) Cramps most often occur at night, perhaps because of reduced blood supply to the muscles. Factors causing cramps are swelling, infection or inflammation, poor circulation, chilling, pregnancy, mineral imbalance, irritation of the muscle or nerves, too much or too little exercise, injury to a muscle, allergy, or microemboli. For some reason not fully understood patients who have had a part of the stomach removed tend to have more frequent muscle cramps. (139)

TREATMENT

1. Better blood circulation will be promoted by a fat-free, sugar free, salt-poor diet.

2. An abundance of green leafy vegetables will insure a good mineral level in the diet.

3. A heating pad applied to the area of cramping may relieve the problem. Some people need alternating hot and cold compresses; apply heat for 6 minutes, and cold for 30 seconds, with four changes.

4. Persons who suffer from leg cramps at night should keep bed covers loose, or use a foot cradle to keep the weight of the covers off the feet. People sleeping on their stomach may extend their feet over the edge of the mattress to maintain a more neutral foot position.

5. Patients with leg cramps should learn to stretch their legs with the feet flexed up, rather than down. (138)

6. An exercise to prevent nighttime cramps was reported in 1979, and we have used it with considerable success. The patient stands with his shoes off, facing a wall 2 to 3 feet away. He leans forward, bracing against the wall with his hands and arms. Keeping the heels on the floor, the patient tilts forward to the wall until a moderate pulling sensation develops in the calf muscles. Hold the stretching position for ten seconds, stand up straight for a five second rest period of relaxation, and repeat the exercise for a total of three stretches. The exercise should be carried out three times daily. Almost half of the patients reported cure of their cramps within three days, and all in the study reported a cure within a week without any further treatment. (140)

7. Leg cramps of pregnancy may be caused by increased pressure from the uterus, fatigue, excessive relaxation due to hormones of pregnancy, chilling, muscle tenseness, etc. Treatment consists of frequent rest periods with the feet elevated, adequate intake of calcium in the diet, and comfortable warm clothing. If a woman develops a cramp she should push the toes upward while applying pressure to the knee to flatten the affected

extremity. This often provides immediate relief. (141) Another exercise is for the woman to lie on her back on a firm surface, with the knees slightly flexed. She extends the knee, straightening and lifting the leg. This is performed twice for each leg. Then, with a knee extended, she moves her ankle around in a complete range of motion for eight rotations. Let that leg rest while the other is rotated, then repeat the procedure. (142)

8. Modified Buerger-Allen exercises may be used. Lie flat on the back in a bed with the feet elevated for two minutes, or until they become blanched. Sit on the edge of the bed with the legs dangling over for three minutes or until the legs become pink. Move the feet up and down, flex the ankles in and out, massage and manipulate the toes, feet, and lower legs. Lie back on the bed, cover with blankets to keep the legs warm, and rest for two minutes. Exercises should be carried out six times each, four times a day.

9. Low back and leg exercises assist in improving circulation to the extremities. Sit on the floor with the legs straight out in front of you, with your feet against the wall. Slowly reach for your toes with your fingers, then sit back slowly. Reach for the left foot with the right hand, then the right foot with the left hand. With hands locked behind the head, twist slowly to the right to touch the left leg with the right elbow. Return to the starting position and twist to the left.

10. Soak in a tub of warm water (100 to 110 degrees F.). Massage the toes, foot, and calves. Soaks should be taken twice daily.

11. Rubbing alcohol massaged in with gentle pressure will improve circulation.

12. Avoid the use of tobacco.

13. Peppermint tea may be helpful in muscle spasms and cramps, and may be applied externally as a compress. Peppermint contains camphorous principles which assist in pain relief. (302)

14. Sleep on a firm mattress with the head of the bed elevated on two inch blocks. If feet swell or the patient has phlebitis, he should elevate the foot of the bed four inches.

15. Elevate legs on a stool when sitting.

16. Do not wear garters or any clothing that constricts the body.

17. Do not sit with crossed legs.

18. Do not stand in one position for hours without moving. Shift the body weight, and move frequently.

19. Get off the feet for five minutes every hour. Take shoes off, and massage feet, exercise toes. (143)

20. Standing on tiptoes will often relieve cramps. (144)

21. Pinch the upper lip between the thumb and index finger as though you were trying to avoid a bad smell. Hold it for 20 or 30 seconds, or until the cramping disappears. (145)

22. Cramps caused by varicose veins or pregnancy may be prevented by elevating the foot of the bed nine inches. When sleeping with one pillow the heart is below the level of the leg veins to encourage drainage. (146)

23. If overweight reduce weight to normal or slightly below normal. (147)

24. Reduce whole milk intake. Eat slowly, and chew your food thoroughly. (147)

OSTEOPOROSIS

Osteoporosis is a decrease in bone tissue which causes weakening of the bone. It is the result of an imbalance between the rate of bone formation and the rate of bone destruction. (405) The most common symptoms are skeletal pain, deformities, and increased susceptibility to fractures.

Approximately 25 to 30% of all white females in the United States develop symptomatic osteoporosis. Although older men between the ages of 50 and 70 may develop osteoporosis it is predominantly a disease of females. Osteoporosis is rare in black males, and less common in black females than in white females. It is more common past the menopause than prior to it.

EXERCISE AND OSTEOPOROSIS

Several studies have shown that physical activity favors bone formation. Some feel that the decline in physical activity as people age may be the principal underlying reason for the high rate of osteoporosis in elderly people. These people suggest that the goal of therapy is to achieve the highest possible bone mass before old age, and to maintain it as long as possible.

G. Donald Whedon, who has served as a consultant to NASA, has observed that even quiet standing for three hours a day had a somewhat positive effect on calcium balance, and four hours of ambulation were sufficient to prevent loss of calcium even if the remaining 20 hours were spent in bed. Dr. Whedon feels that the best exercise for preserving bone mass is gravitational, with active weight-bearing movement such as walking or jogging. (414)

Without gravity the bones begin to lose calcium. During one eight day space trip a group of astronauts lost 200 mg. of calcium per day, despite vigorous exercise programs. The absence of gravity in space makes it impossible to walk, so the bones begin to lose calcium. (432)

Lack of exercise in aging persons may contribute to the development of osteoporosis. The size and density of the skeleton increase with physical stresses.

Bone mass can be increased by strain changes that are well within the range of normal daily activity. The frequency of the strain appears more important than its intensity, suggesting that moderate daily exercise may reverse age-related bone loss. (409)

Intense muscular exercise expands to a significant degree the calcium pool and increases the rate of calcium deposition in the bone. (402)

Bed rest had been shown to be a potent stimulus to bone resorption and induces a negative calcium balance. Localized osteoporosis occurs in bones placed in plaster casts or immobilized by arthritis. These factors show that bones undergo disuse atrophy even in normal hormonal balance. Many years ago physicians noted that hemiplegics had an increased incidence of osteoporosis and fractures on the affected side. They began to refer to this phenomenon as immobilization or disuse osteoporosis.

Chinese and Bantu women, who have a higher level of physical activity, have a lower incidence of osteoporosis than do less active British and Swedish women. Men who exercise regularly have a higher bone density than those who do not exercise regularly.

Forty women, aged 69 to 95, living in a nursing home, were divided into exercising and non-exercising groups. The exercise group exercised lightly to moderately for 30 minutes a day, three days a week. The women in the physical activity program showed less bone loss at the end of the study, and some actually showed an increase in bone formation. (402)

Nine postmenopausal women exercised as a group for one hour a day, three days a week for one year. Nine other women, maintaining their usual amounts of physical activity served as a control group. Both groups continued their usual diets. Total body calcium increased in the exercise group, while it decreased in the control group. (403)

PROTEIN AND OSTEOPOROSIS

The amount of protein a man eats may influence the level of calcium in his body. Tests at the University of Wisconsin reveal that a high-protein diet causes calcium loss. (416) Studies at Fairleigh Dickinson University confirmed this finding. (417)

The American diet is rich in protein due to excessive meat intake. Elderly Eskimos who consume a high-meat diet have significantly lower bone mineral levels than do age-matched Caucasians. (418)

Studies of vegetarians and non-vegetarians in the sixth to ninth decade of life revealed that bone mineral content in meat eaters was decreased 35%, while in the vegetarians it was only 18%. The fact that the changes were not seen in studies of younger vegetarian and non-vegetarian controls suggests that the changes are truly associated with dietary differences.

The high levels of phosphorus in meat may add to the effects of high protein in depriving the body of calcium. Osteoporosis has been produced by feeding animals a high phosphorus diet.

Long-term administration of acid to rats caused osteoporosis, while administration of alkali prevented loss of calcium. Animal proteins and soda pops are high in phosphorus and are known as "acid-ash" foods. (419) Most vegetables and fruits (other than plums, cranberries, and prunes) are "alkaline-ash" foods. (420)

CARBOHYDRATES AND OSTEOPOROSIS

Laboratory animals given a high carbohydrate diet (56% sucrose) in an attempt to induce periodontal disease, were observed to exhibit severe bone disturbances in only six weeks. Sugar apparently contributes to osteoporosis. (421)

CALCIUM AND OSTEOPOROSIS

For years physicians have said that osteoporosis is caused by a lack of dietary calcium, however this theory has not been proven.

Approximately two-thirds of dietary calcium is not absorbed by the body; rather it is excreted in the stool.

A 1973 study revealed no significant differences in bone density between milk drinkers and non-milk drinkers. As a matter of fact, long-bone fractures occurred significantly more often among other milk-drinking osteoporotics than among non milk-drinking osteoporotics. This could suggest that milk drinking is injurious to osteoporotics. (404).

Studies do not show significant correlations between calcium intake and the degree of osteoporosis. (407) Osteoporosis occurs in patients with higher than average calcium intakes, and structural changes in bones have been shown to be unrelated to the level of dietary calcium. (405) Furthermore, decreased intestinal calcium absorption and changes in calcium conservation have been observed in normal men and women 20 to 30 years older than osteoporotic patients. (405) Why did these patients not develop osteoporosis?

Populations taking an average of 300 mg. of calcium a day (less than half of the recommended daily allowance) do not appear deficient in bone formation unless they are also deficient in vitamin D. (406) Prisoners in Peru with calcium intakes of only 0.2 to 0.3 gm. daily were observed to be in metabolic equilibrium. (408)

"If alterations in calcium intake and retention are in any way related to osteoporosis, they most probably represent a contributory rather than a primary cause." (405)

DIETARY FAT AND OSTEOPOROSIS

Nine studies on old rats and hamsters revealed that the loss of calcium was directly related to the level of fat in the diet. The daily loss of calcium of the high fat diet was more than four times as much as on the low fat diet.

The hardness of the fat also influenced the calcium excretion, Feeding tallow induced greater losses than corn oil. (410)

Polyunsaturated margarine apparently leads to some degree of demineralization of bone in growing rats. (411)

SUNSHINE AND OSTEOPOROSIS

Vitamin D is apparently important in the prevention of osteoporosis. Populations taking less than half the recommended daily allowance of calcium do not develop osteoporosis as long as the vitamin D is adequate. (406) There appears to be an inverse relationship between exposure to sunshine and the development of osteoporosis. (412) Vitamin D supplements should not be taken as excess doses of vitamin D taken repeatedly cause bone deterioration. (413)

SMOKING AND OSTEOPOROSIS

One study reports that middle-aged men and women with symptomatic osteoporosis were almost exclusively heavy smokers. (415)

Women smokers experience an earlier menopause because the polycyclic aromatic hydrocarbons found in cigarette smoke destroy oocytes, resulting in ovarian failure. (402)

TREATMENT

1. Patients should sleep on a firm bed to give support to the spine.

2. Avoid overfatigue.

3. Do not lift any heavy object. Small weights should be lifted with both arms to decrease strain on one side of the body. (422)

4. Avoid the use of estrogens. While estrogen therapy initially increases bone formation, it eventually leads to decreased bone formation and lack of response to parathyroid hormone. (423) Estrogen also increases the risk of breast cancer, stroke, and myocardial infarction (heart attack).

5. Use a diet high in fresh raw fruits and vegetables high in vitamin C. A chronic lack of vitamin C may be related to the onset of osteoporosis. (424, 425)

6. Make the environment safe to prevent falls.

7. Exercise to increase muscle tone of trunk flexors and extensors, strengthen muscles and prevent disuse atrophy and further bone demineralization.

8. Daily outdoor exercise provides vitamin D and stimulates osteoblastic cells.

9. Fluoride is felt by some to play an important role in the prevention of osteoporosis. (426) Fluoride is toxic in excessive amounts. As little as 16 mg. of sodium fluoride a day has produced abnormal bone marrow cytology. (427) Fluorides occur

in minute supplies in all foods and water sources. (428)

10. Avoid the use of heparin, (405) corticosteroids, (429) coffee, antacids containing aluminum, cigarettes, and alcohol as these increase calcium requirements. (430)

11. Avoid chilling. Rats exposed to cold stress develop less dense bone. (431)

12. Alcohol consumption decreases bone density and promotes the formation of osteoporosis.

PARKINSON'S DISEASE

Parkinson's disease is a slowly progressive degenerative disease in which there is destruction of nerve cells in the basal ganglia of the brain. (388) The principal signs are tremor at rest, muscle rigidity, bradykinesia (slow or retarded movement), and loss of the postural reflexes. Parkinson's disease is rare before the age of 40 years, and appears less prevalent among Negroes than among whites. (393) Approximately 1 million people in the United States suffer from it. (394) Males suffer from it slightly more frequently than do females.

Parkinson's disease begins slowly, generally with tremor or slowness of movement in one limb. The patient may first notice a loss of skill in the fingers and thumb. Buttoning and unbuttoning clothes, playing the piano, and writing may become more difficult and slower. The symptoms progress to the other limb on the same side, and usually involve the other side after several years. Disability usually does not occur for 10 to 15 years after onset of symptoms.

Death from Parkinson's disease is rare, but death rates are increased because of aspiration pneumonia, urinary tract infections, and various other diseases which the patient is susceptible to because of his Parkinson's disease.

Tremor is an involuntary rhythmic movement of a body part. Tremor at rest is characteristic of Parkinson's disease and usually affects the fingers and hands before the feet. They generally begin on one side and with time progress to the other side. (387)

Decreased facial expression has long been associated with Parkinson's disease. The old physicians used to say the patient wore a "mask." Abnormally decreased muscular movement and rigidity of the facial muscles are felt to be the cause.

The ability to maintain balance may be impaired, probably due to degeneration of the globus pallidus, one of the brain centers.

Parkinson's disease patients may have difficulty swallowing both foods and liquids due to pharyngeal involvement and poor muscle tone in the muscles used in chewing and swallowing.

Patients are often given L-dihydroxyphenylalanine (L-dopa). Levo-dopa is a synthetic compound of dopa. Symptoms of Parkinson's disease are associated with a deficiency of dopamine in the brain, but dopamine apparently does not cross the blood-brain barrier, so levodopa, the metabolic precursor of dopamine must be given. Levodopa is believed to convert to dopamine in the basal ganglia.

Interestingly, vitamin B-6 is known to reverse the effects of levodopa, and patients using levodopa should avoid vitamin prep-arations containing vitamin B-6. (391)

Most patients given levodopa experience side-effects such as nausea, vomiting, insomnia, agitation, and mental confusion. Liver and kidney damage have been reported. (388)

TREATMENT

The personal efforts of the patient with Parkinson's disease are the key to the degree of success with the treatment. There are no means known to halt the progress of the disease, so the overall goal of therapy is to keep the patient functioning independently as long as possible.

Failure to use and exercise muscles leads to the reduction in their size, which brings on the typical symptoms of Parkinson's disease: deformities, drooping of the body, irregular gait, etc. The patient's determination and faithfulness in his exercise routine will go far in slowing progression of the symptoms.

Just as moving water does not freeze, muscles (which are 80% water) will not freeze when kept moving. Every exercise acts toward keeping the muscles useful.

1. Bring the toes up with every step. The heel should be the first portion of the foot to touch the floor when walking. Patients with Parkinson's disease should take large steps and lift the feet as though stepping over objects on the floor.

   At times the feet feel frozen or glued to the floor. Lifting the toes eliminates muscle spasm and frees the feet to continue walking.

2. Keeping the feet 12 to 15 inches apart when walking or turning gives a broader base of balance.

3. To change directions when walking use short steps with feet widely separated. Do not cross one leg over the other while turning. Practice walking a few yards, turning, walking in the opposite direction, and turning for 15 minutes every day. Practice climbing stairs.

4. Swing the arms forcefully when walking, as this loosens arms and shoulders, decreases fatigue, and shifts body weight off the legs.

5. Sitting and rising from a chair should be practiced at least 12 times daily. Sit down slowly with the body bent sharply forward until touching the seat. Rise rapidly to overcome the "pull of gravity." Placing the feet well apart is often helpful. Sometimes putting the feet slightly backward beneath the chair is easier.

6. Neck, shoulder, finger, thigh, knee and ankle muscles are particularly likely to form contractures and special attention should be given to exercising these muscles. It is the contracture of the anterior group of neck muscles which draw the head and shoulders forward in the typical Parkinson stoop. The patient must constantly strive for proper posture with a straight spine, shoulders back, and head up. Stand with the heels, hips, shoulders and head against a wall, pressing in the lower part of the back to reduce the lumbar curve. Try to hold this posture when walking or standing. (390) Practice looking straight ahead when walking instead of looking down at the feet. Sitting with pillows pressed against the upper spine and moving the head backward as far as possible will stretch these muscles.

An overhead pulley helps up to loosen the shoulders. Lift the arms at least a dozen times daily. Rotate the arms upward as far as possible 12 to 15 times a day. Swing the arms vigorously when walking.

To exercise the elbows place the fingers on the shoulder, then straighten the arm. Repeat 12 to 15 times daily. Stretch the fingers at the same time.

Lying face down on a firm surface, lift the head and shoulders five to ten times three times a day.

Bracing the hands against door jams in a doorway, and doing push-aways with the arms strengthens pectoral muscles. Keeping the head erect and the chin retracted during the exercise.

Ankle contractures can be counteracted by putting the feet on a chair or hassock, suspending the knees, for half an hour a day. A stationary bike is an excellent method of preventing hip adduction. Walking in a "goosestep" with legs stiff is a good form of exercise for the ankles and legs.

Typing, playing a piano, working with clay or putty, buttoning and unbuttoning a piece of clothing, etc., all serve as good finger exercises.

7. Any act that is difficult for the patient to perform should be practiced on a daily basis. If putting on a coat or getting out of bed is difficult, the patient should practice it 20 times a day. Acts done repeatedly become much easier. (389)

8. The progress of Parkinson's disease may be slowed by good nutrition, sufficient rest, exercise in fresh air, and other measures to improve general good health.

9. Chest expansion may be decreased because of muscular rigidity, decreasing vital capacity. Deep breathing exercises will mobilize the rib cage, and improve lung capacity and volume. Diaphragmatic breathing should be practiced at all times.

10. Warm bath and massage will help relax muscles and relieve muscle spasms.

11. Frequent rest periods should be taken. The patient is easily fatigued, and frustrated by his symptoms.

12. Rhythmical exercises to music may help to overcome slowness of motion typical of Parkinson's disease. Marching, clapping and calisthenics are suitable.

13. Clothes with front fastenings, zippers or velcro fasteners rather than buttons, elastic waistbands, and slip-on shoes will assist the patient in dressing himself. Tight fitting garments should be avoided. (387)

14. Overweight patients should reduce as excess weight makes movement more difficult. (387)

15. Constipation is often a problem because of poor muscle tone and lack of physical exercise. Patients should drink at least six glasses of water a day, use a high-fiber diet, and exercise out-of-doors daily.

16. The patient should be encouraged to read aloud as a form of speech therapy. If he speaks as he exhales, he will have better voice volume. Singing with forced lip movement will mobilize the facial muscles. Holding a voice sound for five seconds

helps improve facial control and expression vowel sounds seem to be best. Singing the scales helps improve tone inflection. Extending the tongue to the nose and then to the chin develops tongue control.

17. Drooling may occur because of difficulty swallowing. Skin irritation should be treated with frequent wiping and the use of an emollient such as "vaseline milk" (prepared by emulsifying a small lump of vaseline with water). Patients should be instructed to lie on their side to prevent saliva from pooling in the back of the mouth.

18. Parkinson's disease patients often have excessively oily skin and external eye disease is frequent. Greasy scales should be removed from the eyes daily with a moistened Q-tip. Patients should wash their hands before touching their eyes.

19. Bars in the bathroom, and a non-slip bathtub surface will help prevent falls. Throw rugs should be tacked down.

20. Mouth care is important to prevent aspiration of any remaining food particles, as it is often difficult for Parkinson's disease patients to manipulate and swallow food. After each meal he should brush his teeth and rinse his mouth to remove any remaining food particles.

21. Because of the difficulty swallowing many patients suffer from chronic dehydration which increases the likelihood of urinary tract infection. (387) Fluid intake should be adequate to keep the urine almost colorless.

22. The patient should have a firm bed without a pillow to assist in keeping the spine straight. Lying face down also helps. When walking, clasping the hands behind the back will discourage leaning forward. (388)

23. If the patient had difficulty rising from bed, elevating the head of the bed on 4 inch blocks or attaching a knotted rope to the foot of the bed to allow him to pull himself up may be helpful. Movement may be initiated by vigorous rolling or rocking movements.

24. A group of Parkinson's disease patients were given a series of baths of two hours duration at 92 degrees F., six days a week for five weeks. Baths were followed with alcohol rubs or light general massage. The treatments produced improvement in their symptoms. All medications could be stopped. Rigidity and tremor improved. (392)

PEPTIC ULCER

An ulcer is a cavity in the lining and wall of the esophagus, stomach, pylorus, or duodenum. Gastric ulcers are peptic ulcers occurring in the stomach; duodenal ulcers are peptic ulcers occurring in the first 11 inches of the intestine. Duodenal ulcer is found in males about four times as often as in females, (186) and is most frequent in 25 to 40 year olds. Gastric ulcer occurs in males two-and-one half times as often as in females and is most frequently found in the 40 to 55 age group. Duodenal ulcers occur ten times more frequently than gastric ulcers. Five to fifteen percent of the United States population have ulcers, but probably only about half of them are diagnosed. (184) Many ulcers never produce symptoms severe enough to lead to diagnosis. (185) Peptic ulcers apparently have somewhat of a tendency to run in families as they are two to two-and-a-half times more likely to occur if siblings have ulcers. Ulcers tend to flare up during the spring and fall of the year.

Pain located just beneath the breastbone is a typical symptom of ulcer. Pain may radiate to the back in some cases. The pain is often considered to be heartburn, or an empty stomach. The pain appears when the stomach is empty, and is relieved by the intake of food. Some ulcers are not diagnosed until the person vomits blood. Severe ulcers cause pain at night and may awaken the patient at two or three A.M.

TREATMENT

1. Ulcer treatment has changed drastically in the past few years. Frequent feedings, milk intake, and a bland diet are rapidly being discarded. It is now known that the calcium in milk only stimulates acid production rather than decreasing it as was taught for many years. Milk does indeed initially neutralize stomach acid, but then the calcium promotes the secretion of gastrin, a hormone which triggers the release of more acid, giving a rebound effect. (187)

   Acid stimulation is not the only unfavorable result of a Sippy diet (alternating milk and cream and antacids on a regular basis during the waking hours). The incidence of myocardial infarcts (heart attacks) was more than twice as high in a group of ulcer patients treated with the Sippy diet than in two other control groups. It is felt that the butter fat content of the Sippy diet caused the myocardial infarctions. (188)

2. The bland diet is also being discarded, and the patient encouraged to eat whatever foods agree with him. Bland diets do not relieve ulcer pain, nor do they speed healing of ulcers. Not only are they ineffective; as a rule they are poor nutritionally. (189)

3. The presence of any food in the upper gastrointestinal tract is one of the chief stimulants to acid secretion, and reducing the frequency of food intake is far more important than the composition of the food. (191) The six-feeding program can actually be harmful to the patient with an ulcer. The bedtime feeding is particularly dangerous. Gastric acid production is known to follow a circadian rhythm. It normally increases during the day, encouraged by meals, but decreases in the evening, and nearly stops during the night. Gastric acid concentration remains at relatively low levels during the first hour and a half after a meal, even though acid secretion during this time may be as high as eight times normal. About two hours after the meal, the majority of the stomach content has been emptied, and the concentration of gastric acid rises rapidly even though the secretion of acid decreases to about four times normal. This balance is maintained until about four hours after a meal. If an ulcer patient eats a bedtime meal, at 10 or 11 o'clock P.M. the normal circadian rhythm of acid production is disrupted so that high levels of acid are secreted until 2 or 3 A.M. Unfortunately, this is when the patient has the fewest available defenses to cope with the acid load. (190) We recommend a two meal plan, with breakfast around 7 A.M. and dinner at about 1 P.M. with no between-meal snacks. Regularly scheduled meals allow one to take advantage of the rhythmic production of acid. (190)

4. Even antacids are being discarded as they may actually increase acid production. The calcium carbonate nearly doubles the amount of gastric acid in people who suffer from duodenal ulcers. (192) Side-effects of magnesium antacids include diarrhea, potassium deficiency, abnormally high magnesium levels, and iron deficiency. Aluminum based antacids may cause constipation, weakness, anemia, delayed gastric emptying, and perforation of the colon. Calcium-containing antacids may cause milk-alkali syndrome, rebound acidity, and calcium phosphate deposits in the kidney tubules. Sodium in antacids may induce salt and water retention worsening edema and ascites,

hypertension, and cardiac failure. Bicarbonate antacids may induce alkalosis. (210) Other adverse effects of antacids include osteomalacia induced by lack of phosphorus. Aluminum-containing antacids block the absorption of phosphorus, (193) and phosphorus is required for strong bones. While consuming antacids patients absorb up to 20 times less fluoride. (194) Aluminum is currently under scrutiny as a cause of premature senility. Aluminum is retained in the brain and other organs, and scientists believe that excess levels of aluminum are responsible for the increasing incidence of Alzheimer's disease (premature senility) we are currently seeing. (194) Any effective antacid is expected to cause either diarrhea or constipation. (195) Antacids containing sodium bicarbonate could be harmful to the kidneys. (196)

5. Avoid the use of any drugs. Aspirin has long been known to induce gastrointestinal bleeding. A single dose of aspirin tablets is sufficient to induce prolongation of bleeding time, and the effect may persist for up to two days. (197) Alka-seltzer is irritating to the gastric mucosa. Steroids have potent adverse effects, and may increase the incidence of complications. (198)

   It is felt that many drugs (including aspirin) inhibit the synthesis of prostaglandins, and some feel that prostaglandins exert a protective influence of the mucosa. (185)

6. Do not smoke. Smokers have more gastric and duodenal ulcers, a higher death rate from ulcers, and slower healing of their ulcers. Smoking inhibits pancreatic bicarbonate secretion and promotes duodenogastric reflux. (185)

7. Caffeine and caffeine-containing beverages cause a prolonged increase in the stomach acid output. (199) Even decaffeinated coffee stimulates gastric secretion and should not be used.

8. Gastric ulcers may be caused by food stagnation in the stomach. Food stimulates secretion of the hormone gastrin as long as it is in the stomach. Gastrin stimulates excessive production of gastric acid, which in turn leads to ulcers. (200) Eating between meals slows gastric emptying.

9. Chew food properly. Proper mastication mixes urogastrone from the salivary glands with food. Urogastrone protects the intestinal mucosa from erosion in animal tests. (201)

10. Cabbage and several green leafy vegetables contain a factor known as "anti-gizzard erosion factor," later called vitamin U.

It was observed that large amounts of fresh cabbage and lettuce protected guinea pigs from ulcers. The factor was found in the juice of cabbage, thus eliminating the need to eat huge quantities of cabbage. Sixty-two ulcer patients were given at least a liter of cabbage juice daily. The average healing time for seven patients with duodenal ulcer was 10.4 days, compared to 37 days for patients with standard therapy. Six patients with gastric ulcer healed in only 7.3 days, while six patients receiving conventional therapy required 42 days. (203)

The cabbage must be freshly squeezed, and not boiled, as boiling destroys the factor. A mixture of 75% cabbage juice and 25% tomato or celery juice was used with patients who objected to the flavor of the cabbage juice. Raw celery has been found to be high in the factor.

Some patients develop gas, abdominal distress, bloating, and constipation during the first few days of therapy, but after the fifth day of treatment digestive disturbances are rare. (202) If symptoms become severe the juice may be eliminated for a day.

Ordinarily it takes four to five pounds of cabbage to produce one quart of juice. Only fresh, green cabbage should be used. Wilted cabbage contains considerably less factor, and cabbage and cabbage juice held at room temperature for two or three days loses some anti-ulcer potency. Spring, summer, and late summer cabbages are suitable for use, but winter cabbages have very little juice.

Cabbage juice maintains its anti-ulcer activity for at least three weeks if frozen and preserved at approximately 0 degrees C. (202)

The juice may be taken in four or five 6 or 8 ounce servings.

11. Aloe vera gel has been used in the treatment of peptic ulcers with good success. Two to two-and-a-half fluid drams of gel appears to be an effective dose. The author recommends that after healing of the ulcer, patients continue taking a single tablespoonful of aloe vera gel at bedtime. His group of patients had no ulcer recurrences after 18 months of follow-up. Apparently the gel inhibits the secretion of hydrochloric acid. (204)

12. A diet high in sugar stimulates acid production. A high sugar diet for only two weeks drove stomach acid levels up by 20 percent in a group of healthy volunteers. (205)

13. White bread seems to act the same way tobacco does in the production of ulcers. The researchers who did the study felt that whole-grain bread might be of benefit to ulcer patients. (206)

14. Dr. Maxwell Berry of Emory University reported to the 1956 meeting of the American College of Gastroenterology that 75% of peptic ulcer patients also have the hypoglycemic syndrome. He stated that there was tremendous acid production in the stomachs of patients with low blood sugar. He feels that a very large percentage of people with the hypoglycemic syndrome will develop ulcers. (207) Any problem with blood sugar should be treated.

15. Potatoes are often very helpful to peptic ulcer patients. Vitamin C has an important healing influence on wounds, and potatoes are high in vitamin C. Furthermore, potatoes have an alkaline reaction, assisting in acid neutralization. Two or more potato feedings daily may be helpful. (208) Potatos may be baked, boiled, mashed, etc., but should not be fried, and milk should not be added.

16. Dried sweet almonds, well-chewed, raise the pH of the gastric juice, decrease hydrochloric acid production, and significantly inhibit peptic activity. (209)

17. Ripe olives are known to be soothing to the stomach. Four to six olives may be taken with meals. Use only black or green ripe olives; avoid those canned in vinegar.

18. Millet is soothing to the gastrointestinal tract, and is usually well tolerated by peptic ulcer patients.

19. Attention should be paid to dress. The extremities should be well clothed to balance the circulation and avoid congestion in the abdomen.

20. Remember that exercise neutralizes stress. Have a regular program of out-of-door exercise daily.

21. For peptic ulcer pain apply an ice bag to the abdomen just above the navel or to the portion of the spine between the shoulder blades. (275)

POISON IVY

Poison ivy grows either as a climbing vine or upright shrub. The leaves grow in clusters of three, one to the tip of the stalk, and the other two opposite each other. The sticky sap contains urushiol, a combination of plant resin and volatile oil, which can cause an allergic skin reaction.

Urushiol must come in contact with the skin directly or indirectly. Clothing, tools, and pets may carry the urushiol to the unsuspecting victim. Even dead roots and stems contain urushiol, and smoke from burning plants may carry droplets of it to the skin, or into the nose, throat and lungs. (24) Sensitivity to the toxin varies from person to person, and may vary from period to period in a person's life.

Anyone working with poison ivy should wear protective clothing, including gloves. Clothing should be washed promptly as the resin can remain on the clothing for several days after exposure. An alkaline laundry soap or detergent should be used to wash the body if one inadvertently comes in contact with poison ivy, preferably shortly after the exposure. The oil may be spread from place to place on the body by scratching before washing.

Reactions to poison ivy vary from redness and itching to blister formation and edema, which may be followed by a secondary infection. (25) Reaction may begin within six hours, or be delayed several days after exposure.

TREATMENT

1. Calamine lotion without additives may help relieve itching.

2. Wet dressings or soaks are comforting and may prevent secondary infection. A solution of physiologic saline (2 level teaspoons of salt to a quart of water) is excellent for this. Saturate clean cloths (old bed sheeting is satisfactory), wring out until it does not drip, and apply several layers on and around the affected area. Change the compress every three to four minutes for an hour, remove compress for an hour, and repeat the process through the waking hours.

3. Jewelweed has been reported useful in the treatment of poison ivy, but one study showed that areas treated with water alone, and those not treated both responded better than those treated with jewelweed. (26)

4. Plantain leaf has been reported to bring rapid relief in cases of itching. (27)

5. Some people have good results with lemon juice. Wash the exposed area with lemon juice, pat (don't wipe) dry, and apply

as much lemon juice as possible. If symptoms return, repeat the process.

6. Salt may be wet and rubbed on the affected area. It burns a bit, but is helpful to some.

7. Vinegar is reported useful if used in the same way as lemon juice.

8. Running hot water (as hot as can be tolerated without burning oneself) over the area will often stop the itch and give several hours of relief. Repeat the treatment as needed. (28)

9. Goldenseal tea may be used as a wash or compress for poison ivy. (293) A paste may be made from the powdered root. (295)

10. Blend oatmeal into a fine powder, and add a small amount of water to make a paste to soothe poison ivy. (294)

11. The juice of aloe vera is soothing to poison ivy blisters. (295)

12. Avoid over-the-counter poison ivy preparations. Dr. Albert Kligman, a world authority on poison ivy reports that not one of 34 popular poison ivy remedies tested was more effective than water or calamine lotion. Furthermore, many of these products may produce an allergic reaction. (521)

13. Banana peels rubbed directly on the area bring relief for as long as four hours.

PRURITUS ANI

Pruritus ani is manifested by itching around the anus. It is actually a symptom of a disease, rather than a disease itself. (31) It is seen in men about four times as often as in women. (29) Causes are poor hygiene, infection, skin diseases such as psoriasis, eczema, and seborrheic dermatitis, parasites, estrogen deficiency, diabetes, liver disease, and contact dermatitis in response to perfumed or dyed toilet tissue, soap, deodorants, underclothing, etc.

TREATMENT

1. Elimination of moisture is the major goal in therapy. Moisture, fecal soiling, and leakage are primary factors in many cases of pruritus ani.

2. Avoid the use of anesthetic medications with "caine" in the name as they may produce an intense allergic reaction and

make the condition much worse. They also tend to be moisture-holding and perpetuate the problem. (29)

3. A number of foods have been shown to cause allergies which lead to itching. These include beer and other alcoholic beverages, milk, coffee, tea, cola drinks, citrus fruits and juices, tomatoes, chocolate, nuts, popcorn, and highly seasoned and spicy foods. (29, 33)

4. Avoid the use of any drug. Many drugs irritate the colon and precipitate pruritus.

5. Do not use mineral oil as a laxative. The oil may seep out of the rectum.

6. Avoid the use of milk and all milk-containing foods. Milk is a constipating food and it is often difficult to pass the pasty stool. Patients with lactose intolerance have frequent liquid movements, necessitating frequent wiping of the area, which may produce trauma to the skin of the area. This is also true of patients with dumping syndrome, malabsorption syndrome, and chronic diarrhea. Leakage adds moisture and irritants to the area.

7. Trauma to the skin is probably the second most common cause of pruritus ani. Frequent or vigorous wiping, as well as scratching may cause the skin to weep, adding more moisture to the area. Adult athletes are very prone to pruritus, probably because of frequent showering after physical activity and perhaps the overuse of soap.

8. High-strung, nervous individuals seem to be more susceptible than the average person. Adopt a lifestyle that will minimize stress.

9. Pinworms are rarely the cause of pruritus ani in the adult, but may be the sole cause in children.

10. A tub or sitz bath morning and afternoon will be helpful in relieving symptoms. Add one-half to one ounce of Purex or Clorox to the water.

11. Avoid the use of soap in the anal area, as soap is highly alkaline, and may alter the normal acidity of the skin. A mild irritation is set up when the alkaline fluid comes in contact with the acid skin. (30)

12. After bowel movements, wet tissue or cotton should be used to clean the area. Do not leave a wet dressing against the skin.

Pat—don't rub—the area dry. One may use a hair dryer to assist in drying. Above all, don't scratch!

13. An irrigation of the anal skin using a 3 or 4 ounce bulb syringe of warm water may be helpful if the itching is worse after a bowel movement. This will assist in cleansing the area. Be careful to dry thoroughly after the irrigation.

14. A thin pledget of dry cotton may be worn during the day to absorb discharges. This should be taken from the side of the roll of cotton, and should be thin enough that you do not notice it is in place. It may be dusted with cornstarch. Do not use a cotton ball. The pledget should be changed frequently during the day.

15. Avoid the use of tight underclothing and such things as girdles which increase local perspiration and tend to retain moisture, inducing itching. Cotton fabrics evaporate moisture and are better than synthetic fabrics. (32)

16. A warm (not hot) goldenseal tea bag may be applied to the area for up to one-half hour to relieve itching.

17. Avoid gas-forming foods.

18. A cream containing the "cooling" counter-irritants such as menthol, camphor, and eucalyptus may be very helpful to relieve itching. One such is Soltice, which has a vanishing cream base (not petrolatum which is greasy). Try a small area first, as it may be too strong.

RAYNAUD'S PHENOMENON

Raynaud's phenomenon is characterized by an intermittent decrease in blood flow to the extremities, generally the hands, but the feet and toes, nose, cheeks, ears, and chin may also be involved. (137) The afflicted body parts may initially blanch due to spasm of the blood vessels, then change to bright red as the blood vessels distend, bringing increased blood into the area. The fingers may initially feel numb and cold, then begin tingling, swelling, and become painful.

Raynaud's phenomenon may be due to various systemic disorders, or it may be primary, in which case it is called Raynaud's disease. Raynaud's disease occurs mostly in women, while Raynaud's phenomenon is seen about equally in both sexes. The disease usually begins in the teens or early twenties, but onset may occur at any time. The phenomenon tends to occur later, generally after the age of 30. Symptoms in the phenomenon may be one-sided, while in the disease the symptoms are generally bilateral and symmetrical. (157)

Attacks may occur several times a day, or they may be relatively rare. Mild cases usually last only a few minutes; severe cases may persist several hours. The hands generally appear normal between attacks, but if the disease is advanced and severe, they may remain slightly bluish. With the advance of the disease, the attacks become more frequent and last longer. Because of lack of blood in the area, the fingers become swollen and the skin becomes pale or discolored, shiny, taut, and smooth. The nails may become clubbed and deformed. There may be decreased sensation, with awkwardness of fine movement. There may be recurrent infections and gangrene.

TREATMENT

1. Attacks are provoked by chilling. Dress warmly at all times, being careful to keep the extremities as well covered as the trunk, to assure even distribution of blood. In cold weather, clothing should be of a type that will retain body heat by trapping it in layers of air. Tightly woven, thick wool socks and mittens will greatly reduce heat loss from the hands. Mittens are better than gloves, as gloves allow the cold air to surround and take up heat from each finger.

2. The feet should be kept warm with fleece-lined footwear, or innersoles made of a reflective material. Hands and feet should be warm before putting on footwear or mittens. After the fingers or toes are cold it generally requires an external source of heat to reheat them.

3. Stress often induces Raynaud's phenomenon by causing spasm of the blood vessels. Adopt a lifestyle free from stress as far as possible. Vigorous out-of-door exercise daily is recommended. Remember that exercise neutralizes stress.

4. Downhill skiers use the following technique to warm cold hands: Hold the hands above the head, permitting the venous blood to drain from the hands. Whirl the arms, driving arterial blood into the capillaries by centrifugal force. In 1978 Dr. Donald McIntyre reported success in aborting Raynaud's attacks by having the patient briskly swing the affected extremity

in the way that a softball pitcher would move the arm (downward behind the body, up in front of the body) in a continuous 360 degree movement. He placed emphasis on the downward sweep so as to combine both centrifugal and gravitational forces in the blood vessels communicating with the outstretched fingers. This maneuver increases intraarterial pressure to the extent that it counteracts the vasoconstricting action of the smooth muscles. (166) Anyone can observe the reddening effect in one hand as compared with the opposite. This maneuver was picked up by other physicians who also used it successfully, but some patients with back problems were reporting lumbar discomfort after the maneuver. It was discovered that having the patient swing his arm in the arc in front of the body, rather than to the side of the body, was just as successful, and caused no lumbar discomfort. The upward motion should be in front of the trunk; the downward motion to the side. (167)

5. Avoid contact with cold objects, even for split seconds. During meal preparation, wash vegetables in tepid, not cold water. Use mittens to remove cold items from the refrigerator or freezer.

6. Central heat is helpful as it keeps all rooms in the house at approximately the same temperature. Avoid sudden changes in room temperature when moving about the house.

7. Electric blankets and heated water beds keep the patient from getting chilled at night.

8. When out-of-doors, face into the sun rather than away from it. This helps to keep the entire body warmer.

9. Immersion of the affected part in warm (not hot) water no warmer than 90 degrees F. will hasten relief. Because of decreased blood flow in the area one needs to be cautious to avoid burning the tissues. Some patients report better success in warming the backs of the hands and upper chest and backs of the shoulders first. One may warm these areas by the use of a heating pad, a hot water bottle, a warm shower, or tub bath, or a warm washcloth applied to the area.

10. A warm drink also seems to help in warming some patients.

11. One lady reported that having her hands and fingers massaged every evening reduced the frequency and severity of the attacks. Massage apparently stimulates circulation to the area.

12. Smoking should be avoided, as tobacco causes constriction of the blood vessels. (158) Even "passive" smokers, people who do not themselves smoke, but are around others who do, may develop Raynaud's. One 47-year-old woman, married to a heavy smoker for two-and-one-half years developed Raynaud's. The man's former wife also had Raynaud's which cleared up within six months of their divorce. The second wife's symptoms cleared in two weeks after her husband cut down on smoking, and stopped smoking in the room where his wife was. The husband also had Raynaud's but could not be persuaded to stop smoking. (161) Passive inhalation of nicotine has been shown to decrease cutaneous blood flow, and increase vascular resistance. (162)

13. Avoid the use of drugs. They are of questionable benefit at best, and most Raynaud patients find that the side-effects of the commonly used medications outweigh the benefits and would rather endure the symptoms of the disease. (157) A number of drugs are known to induce Raynaud's phenomenon (159) including ergot, beta blocking drugs, cytotoxic agents, and birth control pills.

14. Avoid activities that involve vibration of the hands. In one study 50% of a group of pneumatic percussion drillers had Raynaud's phenomenon, compared to 5.6% of the general population. (159) Stone cutters, rivet drivers, metal grinders, and chain saw operators have higher rates of Raynaud's than do other occupations. (160) Repeated trauma to the hands caused by occupations such as carpentry, mechanics, lathe operators, and many laborers may also induce severe Raynaud's phenomenon. (160) Using an electric typewriter and having adequate heating in the winter will be beneficial to secretaries.

15. Birth control pills have been implicated as a cause of Raynaud's phenomenon. The symptoms improve after the use of birth control pills is discontinued.

16. Use a fat-free, sugar-free diet. Patients with Raynaud's phenomenon have been shown to have increased viscosity of the blood, and an increased amount of aggregation (clumping together) of the red blood cells, (163, 164) which may play an important part in decreasing blood flow to affected areas. Sugar increases triglycerides (fatty substances) in the blood.

17. Keep well hydrated at all times to improve circulation. Drink plain water, not highly sweetened soft drinks, teas, coffee, or even fruit juices.

18. Abstain from alcoholic beverages, highly seasoned foods, and use a low protein diet. (165)

19. Sunbaths may be helpful in improving general physical resistance to disease. Ultraviolet rays are essentially a blood tonic due to chemical changes in the blood. (165)

RESTLESS LEG SYNDROME

Restless leg syndrome is an annoying sensation of discomfort in the legs, generally between the knees and feet, which makes the victim feel that he must move his legs. It is often described as pain, itching, cramping, restlessness, twitching, crawling, or aching. It occurs most often shortly after going to bed, but may occur after sitting still for a long period of time. Many people complain of loss of sleep because they must get out of bed and walk to relieve the sensation. After a period of time the symptoms abate and the patient may sleep, but a little later the symptoms may recur. This may happen a number of times during the night. (43) Five percent of people suffer restless leg syndrome, women more than men, and older people more than young. (40) Its cause is unknown, but studies have suggested a relationship to various factors including gastrectomy, diabetes, uremia, (40) motion sickness remedies, pregnancy, hereditary factors, prostatitis, pulmonary disease, iron deficiency, carcinoma, exposure to cold (42) and stress. Mild weakness of the legs may also be present. (41)

TREATMENT

1. Eliminate the use of caffeine and all caffeine-containing products. ". . . caffeine is the major etiological factor in the causation of the restless leg syndrome." (43)

2. Lying face down has brought relief to some patients. (44)

3. Use a diet high in foods containing folic acid and vitamin E (47) as these have been shown in some studies to be helpful. Foods high in folic acid are beans, potatoes, dark green leafy vegetables, asparagus, broccoli, lima beans, peanuts, beets, cabbage, lettuce, and avocados. Vitamin E is found in wheat germ,

wholemeal cereals, broccoli, leafy vegetables, and vegetable oils. (45, 46)

4. A warm soaking bath before bedtime is often helpful. After getting out of the tub, dry off briskly, dress warmly, and go to bed. Do not allow the bare feet to touch a cold floor. Some people find wearing knee socks helpful, others find they are unable to sleep with them on.

5. An occasional person reports relief with cold sponging of the legs. (40)

6 Avoid overusing the legs. The syndrome seems to be worsened with strenuous exercise. (41)

7. A significant number of cases may be due to venous stasis. (547) Elastic stockings or bandages may prevent stagnation of blood in the leg veins. Do not cross the legs. Lie down periodically during the day to elevate and rest the legs.

8. Women should avoid narrowly pointed shoes and thin high heels.

9. Rotating the feet for a few minutes may relieve symptoms.

10. A low salt diet may be helpful.

RHEUMATOID ARTHRITIS

Rheumatoid arthritis is a chronic disease of unknown cause. Symptoms include joint pain, stiffness, swelling, redness, heat, deformity, and limitation of motion. Fatigue, anemia, weight loss, and fever may also be present. It is two to three times more frequent in women than in men. It most commonly occurs between the ages of 35 and 45, but may occur at any age. Stress, physical or mental, is often associated with the onset of the disease, (258) as are exposure, overwork, or acute infections. About five million people in the United States have rheumatoid arthritis.

Some patients have only a brief period of illness lasting only a few months, followed by months or even years of remission. Permanent remission occasionally occurs. The likelihood of remission is greater early in the course of the disease. Each attack seems to be worse than those preceding it.

Vague pain, stiffness, weight loss, numbness and tingling of the hands and feet may precede the onset of rheumatoid arthritis.

The joints of the hands, elbows, knees, and ankles are most commonly involved.

In about 10 to 15% of rheumatoid arthritis cases the disease progresses to the point that they are confined to a bed or wheelchair. (258)

TREATMENT

1. A low-fat diet has proven helpful to rheumatoid arthritis patients. (See Appendix C.) Dr. Charles Lucas of Wayne State University School of Medicine says that debilitating pain and severe joint swelling are virtually eliminated by a strict low-fat diet. When the patients went off the low-fat diet their symptoms returned. (259)

2. Fasting can bring temporary relief from rheumatoid arthritis, but pain, swelling and stiffness of the joints return a few days after the fast is broken. (260)

3. In 1949 a hypoallergenic diet was found to be helpful in rheumatoid arthritis. A 1981 study (261) revealed that 86% of a group of rheumatoid arthritics had onset of rheumatic symptoms in response to allergies. Some patients were found to be sensitive to as many as ten different things. Soy products, milk, egg, coffee and sugar were common offenders. A trial on a diet free of the most common allergens (Appendix A) may be quite beneficial.

   Dr. R. Shatin of Victoria, Australia feels that a predisposition to rheumatoid arthritis is linked with gluten sensitivity. He points out that population groups that use large quantities of wheat, rye, and oats in their dietary also have high rates of rheumatoid arthritis. (266)

   Nightshades may play a role in the development of rheumatoid arthritis. For a discussion of this see Arthritis.

4. Many arthritics are known to have anemia, but this should be treated with a diet high in iron-rich foods. One 49-year-old woman reported that her symptoms worsened when she took ferrous sulphate (the iron preparation commonly given for anemia). She was hospitalized and preliminary tests done to measure such things as joint pain and grip strength. After three days of oral iron supplements she had a twofold rise in joint pain, increased morning stiffness (from 15 minutes to 60 minutes) and a 30% decrease in grip strength. (262)

5. A study carried out at Addenbrookes Hospital in Cambridge, England, revealed that joint lesions could be induced in rabbits by giving them cow's milk to drink. (263)

   One patient was demonstrated to have flare-ups of her rheumatoid arthritis with the intake of milk and cheese. Excluding these items from her diet produced a considerable improvement. (263) Three weeks after eliminating these foods she began to feel better and eventually morning stiffness completely resolved and the inflammation almost completely disappeared. On one occasion she inadvertently ate dairy produce and her symptoms returned within 12 hours.

   A most interesting study relating milk and rheumatoid arthritis comes from Stockholm, Sweden. Nanna Svartz, of the King Gustaf V Research Institute says that the primary cause of rheumatoid arthritis is an infection and the infectious agent exists in milk. (264) Diplostreptococcus agalactiae (DSA) can be isolated from the nasopharynx of 75 to 80% of rheumatoid arthritis patients compared to only 20% of persons with other diseases, or healthy persons. DSA are highly resistant to heat and are able to withstand pasteurization temperatures. DSA was found in all specimens of milk from Sweden that were examined.

6. That rheumatoid arthritis may be viral in origin is also suggested by the fact that during the five year period prior to the onset of rheumatoid arthritis, rheumatoid arthritis patients had a greater exposure to dogs, cats, birds, and sick animals than did a similar group of control patients. (265)

7. One group of rheumatoid arthritics were given a diet of raw fruits and vegetables for a two week period with most gratifying results. After the two week period cooked foods were reintroduced with continued improvement. No salt was added to any of the food, raw or cooked, and all food was prepared fresh for every meal. (267)

8. Exercise is the most important single part of the physical therapy program in rheumatoid arthritis. Exercise assists in maintaining optimum levels of function, prevents and corrects deformities, controls pain, and strengthens weakened muscles. Exercise can actually relieve pain; continuous immobilization can cause increasing pain.

   The proper balance between rest and exercise is essential as overactivity can inflame affected joints. Fatigue is a common symptom and tolerance to exercise must be carefully evaluated. The patient may experience some pain for a short time with exercise, but pain which persists for several hours after exercise may indicate excessive exercise. (258)

A weight and pulley system may be used for elbows and shoulders; bicycle riding increases mobility of the hips and knees.

The following simple exercises should be carried out daily. Initially do each exercise five times, increase as tolerance permits:

A. Make a fist, then straighten fingers.

B. Rotate wrists in a complete circle.

C. Bend and straighten arms.

D. Raise hand to shoulder, then straighten arm to side.

E. Raise hand to shoulder, then straighten to front of body.

F. Bend and straighten legs.

G. Lying on your back, lift one leg at a time.

H. Lying on your stomach, lift one leg at a time.

I. Still lying face down, lift head and shoulders.

J. Swing legs over side of bed. (268)

Exercises may be performed more effectively if preceded by the application of heat.

Exercises should be carried out slowly and smoothly.

9. Bed rest is important in acute rheumatoid arthritis. The more acute the disease or the greater number of joints involved, the greater the benefit of bed rest. Complete bed rest is anti-inflammatory. Two or four hours of rest during the day may be adequate for mild rheumatoid arthritis. The bed must be firm in order for bedrest to be effective, and the patient must be correctly positioned. Pillows should not be placed under the knees, as that position encourages knee flexion contractures. Hip flexion contractures are prevented by having the patient lie face down for 30 minutes two to three times a day. It is better not to use a pillow, but if the patient insists only a small pillow or folded towel should be allowed. A small pillow under the ankles will tend to straighten the knees. Small pillows or folded towels may be placed under the elbows or wrists to straighten the arms. Hands should be positioned with the palms up.

10. Overweight patients should lose weight to reduce strain on the weight-bearing joints.

11. Work on maintaining correct posture at all times. Pain and swelling encourage a position of deformity which increases the work load of the muscles.

12. Stretch nylon gloves worn at night help to keep hands warm and relieve numbness and tingling of the fingers.

13. An electric blanket at night may decrease morning stiffness. A number of people report that sleeping in a sleeping bag accomplishes the same thing.

14. A warm tub bath or shower in the morning reduces morning stiffness.

15. Moist heat applications for 15 to 30 minutes twice a day will reduce muscle spasm and stiffness. They are particularly beneficial if applied just prior to exercise periods. A hot shower often serves well. Heat makes tendons more flexible and for some unknown reason lowers the temperature of the synovial fluid.

    Moist heat penetrates tissues slightly better than dry heat, but the body tolerates dry heat at higher temperatures than moist heat.

    When a joint is acutely inflamed with redness and swelling, ice packs will relieve swelling and pain and assist in restoring function. Crushed ice in a plastic bag laid over the joint will often provide striking pain relief.

16. Deep breathing exercises are helpful to patients with rheumatoid arthritis. (258)

17. Massage may relieve pain and muscle aches. Actively inflamed joints should not be massaged as massage may aggravate inflammation. Massage should be over surrounding muscles, not over joints. (258)

18. Some patients prefer ice massage of painful joints rather than hot. (269)

19. Alternating hot and cold baths have been shown to be excellent in rheumatoid arthritis. (270) Six minutes for the hot applications and four minutes for the cold bring a significant increase in blood flow in the area.

20. Paraffin baths as described under "Gout" are also very beneficial. Paraffin raises skin temperature more readily than other
measures.

21. Aloe vera gel has been reported successful in relieving pain in
rheumatic joints. (303)

SINUSITIS

Sinusitis is an inflammation of the sinuses. A sinus is an open cavity; the human skull contains eight sinus cavities.

The most common causes of sinusitis are infection and allergies.
Infection from colds, flu, etc., spread easily from the nose because
of their direct continuity into the sinuses. Nose blowing, sneezing,
swimming, and diving during an upper respiratory infection may
hasten the spread of the infection. (370)

The nasal mucus contains lysozyme, a powerful antibacterial
agent which makes the epithelium of the nose and sinuses quite
resistant to infection. Such things as tobacco smoke, alcohol, many
medications, and infection decrease the effectiveness of the body's
natural protective system and predispose the patient to sinus infections. (370)

True sinusitis is not as common as television advertisements
would have us think. Out of every 100 patients who go to an otola-
ryngologist because of "sinus trouble", fewer than ten actually
have sinusitis. (371)

Symptoms of sinusitis are nasal obstruction and discharge, headache, lack of appetite, nausea, cough, sore throat, swelling and
pain over the sinuses involved. The patient may have a low-grade
fever, but with severe infection it may rise as high as 104 degrees F.
(371)

Maxillary sinusitis pain is usually located in the upper teeth and
cheek, but eye pain may be present. The discomfort generally begins in late morning and clears by late afternoon on a daily basis.

When the frontal sinuses are involved, frontal headaches most
severe between 8:00 A.M. and 5:00 P.M. are common.

A constant dull pain behind the eyes suggests ethmoid sinusitis.
there may also be sensitivity to light, pain on eye movements, tearing, and sometimes sore throat and nighttime cough. (370)

TREATMENT

1. Smoking irritates the mucous membranes and inhibits the body's natural cleansing system in the nose, and should be avoided. (371)

2. Avoid cold, damp conditions and chilling as these induce vasoconstriction, lower leukocyte response, and impair phagocytic capabilities predisposing to infections. (372)

3. Maintain a constant room temperature as temperature changes aggravate sinusitis. (373) Air conditioning seems to aggravate sinusitis.

4. A humidity of 40 to 50% will increase comfort. (373)

5. Adequate fluid intake encourages sinus drainage. (371)

6. A room vaporizor may facilitate drainage. (373)

7. Avoid the use of nose drops as they may induce a rebound effect. (371) Vasoconstrictors are used to reduce nasal congestion. Used too frequently or over too long a period of time they become ineffective and may actually worsen the condition. Engorgement is controlled by the autonomic nervous system. Vasoconstrictors stimulate sympathetic nerves, inducing a compensatory relaxation of the vessels of the turbinates after the effects of the nose drops wear off. This relaxation produces nasal stuffiness, causing the nose to be more stuffy than it was before. It takes two or three weeks without the use of nose drops before the reflexes return to normal.

8. Heat over the sinuses often relieves pain. Hot wet compresses, a heat lamp, a 60 watt incandescent light such as a shop lamp, or heating pad may be used.

9. Sniffing warm salt water up into the nose may wash the excess mucus out. Add one-fourth teaspoon of salt to eight ounces of water. It will cause some people to sneeze which will assist in clearing the nose. The use of "Dr. Grossan's nasal irrigator" a commercially available device which fits on a Waterpik and utilizes warm saline, is a very efficient method of irrigating nasal and pharyngeal passages. A bulb syringe from the pharmacy can be utilized as an alternative.

10. Several exercises are valuable in sinusitis. Do them twice a day.

    A. Lie across your bed, face down, with the upper body hanging over the side. Rest your head and lower arm on the floor. Lie face down for three minutes, turn on your left side for three minutes, then on the right side for three minutes. Return to the face down position and cough gently. Hold your breath after each cough for a few seconds, then inhale gently.

B. Sit with your head between your knees. Cough gently as though clearing your throat. Hold your breath for a few minutes to let the mucus drain, then gently inhale.

C. Tap your chest in a regular pattern from the bottom of your chest up toward the neck, and back again, using the fingertips of both hands. Have a helper do the same on your back while you tap the front.

11. Peppermint tea may be helpful to open up the passageways. Some people like a peppermint leaf compress over the affected sinuses. (374)

12. Swimming and diving may wash nasal infection into sinuses, and should be avoided if one has any type of infection. (375) Air travel may act similarly. Avoid flying during respiratory tract infections. Sudden changes in altitude may produce sudden swelling, hemorrhage and pain within the sinus. (375)

13. Allergic rhinitis is a common cause of sinusitis. (375) Avoid any substance you know or suspect allergy to.

14. Some people prefer cold applications to the sinuses rather than hot. Crushed ice may be sealed in a plastic bag and the bag wrapped in a slightly moist towel and applied over the painful sinuses. Put the feet in a hot foot bath at the same time. The cold decreases the flow of blood in the congested sinus membranes, while the hot foot bath draws the blood to the feet. (376)

15. A hot foot bath by itself is often very effective in opening up nasal passages. Keep the feet in the hot water for 20 to 30 minutes. Conclude the treatment by a brief cold water pour to the feet. Rest in bed after the treatment until sweating stops. The treatment may be done several times a day.

16. A hot compress applied to the face is often effective in opening up nasal passages. Squeeze a towel from hot water and apply to a painful area for five minutes, then squeeze a towel from ice water and apply it for 30 seconds. Repeat three times, ending with the cold.

17. Fasting may be quite helpful, although initially symptoms may be worse because of the increased rate of release of toxins.

Fever-inducing baths and hot foot baths will help control symptoms.

18. Six charcoal tablets taken between meals twice daily will assist in the removal of toxins from the body.

19. Garlic tea, made by boiling four cups of water, removing from heat and adding crushed garlic cloves, is reported to relieve stuffiness.

TENNIS ELBOW

Tennis elbow usually presents as tenderness and pain in the elbow and weakness of the hand. The weakness is due to discomfort when gripping objects, not to true muscle weakness.

Tennis elbow occurs more often in non-athletes than in athletes. Housewives, factory workers, golfers, carpenters, and politicians doing a lot of handshaking are all prone to it.

TREATMENT

1. Rest for three or four days is essential. Rest does not mean total immobilization as immobilization leads to muscle atrophy; rest means elimination of the activities that cause pain. (493)

2. Ice may be applied for 30 to 90 minutes daily, depending on the severity of the pain. (493) Some patients find heat more soothing, particularly after the first few days.

3. Avoid cortisone injections as they may cause tendon atrophy or actually dissolve the tendon. (493)

4. Rest alone is generally not adequate to cure tennis elbow. Exercise is very important and will help to prevent recurrences. A hand gripper may be used five to ten minutes four times a day. The elbow should be straight, and the wrist bent to stretch the extensor tendons and aid in strengthening fibrous tendons. (492)

5. Vigorously rubbing the elbow and forearm may be helpful. (494)

6. Fourteen of eighteen patients on a four to five week program of resistive exercise received complete pain relief. (495) Place the arm on a table, palm down, gripping a three pound dumbbell. Flex the wrist upward with a slight radial deviation, and

hold for five seconds. Return to the starting position and rest three seconds. Increase the weight one pound when the exercise can be performed 15 times with ease. Continue increasing weight until eight to ten pounds can be lifted without pain. This generally requires four to six weeks of daily exercise.

To strengthen the forearm rotators start with the arm downward and rotate the forearm 180 degrees, bringing the palm upward and the dumbbell into the horizontal position. Repeat each exercise 15 times. (496)

7. An isometric exercise is reported to prevent tennis elbow. (497) Attempt a backhand swing while holding the throat of the racket with the non-playing hand. Gradually increase the strength of the pull.

8. Many players report relief by placing a band several inches wide around the forearm near the elbow and another just above the wrist. Be certain the bands are not so tight that they interfere with blood flow. (494)

9. A racket with a larger grip, or a lighter racket, not too tightly strung, may help. Some aluminum or fiberglass rackets may cause less pain than wooden ones. (494) Rubbing or warming the arm just prior to playing may increase pain tolerance limits.

THROMBOPHLEBITIS SEE VENOUS THROMBOSIS

THRUSH

Candida albicans, a yeast, is the cause of thrush. The disease is characterized by white patches on the cheeks, tongue, and palate. (15) The small white flakes look like coagulated milk, but unlike milk curds, they cannot be wiped off. If scraped off they usually leave bleeding points. (19) Spores of Candida lodge between the epithelial cells of the mouth and generally separate the layers. The infection then spreads to the surface of the mucous membrane, and gradually spreads. (16) Thrush occurs in approximately 4% of infants; (18) the average length of time from birth to the development of thrush is eight to nine days. (17) Thrush occurs in healthy infants in the neonatal period, but may occur in children and adults whose health is poor.

Infants of diabetic mothers are especially susceptible to thrush because the high glucose level in the mother's urine encourages the growth of the yeast. (15) Infants with cleft lip or palate often develop persistent thrush.

In most cases the disease is self-limiting, (14) clears up readily, and leaves no scars.

It is felt that the most common cause of thrush in the newborn is infection during birth, but the disease may be spread by other patients, from contaminated hands, feeding equipment, and bedding.

TREATMENT

1. Rubber nipples and all objects coming in contact with the baby's mouth should be clean. It the baby is bottle-fed, boil nipples and bottles at least 20 minutes after a thorough washing as the spores are heat resistant. (15)

2. Children with thrush should be isolated from other children.

3. Avoid antibiotics and steroids (20) as these destroy the competing bacteria and allow the Candida to overgrow. Swabbing the infant's mouth with the mother's saliva establishes a competitive flora, and may cut down on the growth of Candida. (21)

4. Give plain water to cleanse the mouth after every feeding. (22)

5. Inspect the mouth before every feeding for the presence of thrush and begin treatment at the first indication.

6. Swab the infected areas with a saturated solution of baking soda three or four times a day.

7. Garlic solution may be swabbed on the lesions several times a day as Candida has been shown to be sensitive to garlic. (23)

ULCERATIVE COLITIS

Ulcerative colitis is an inflammatory disease which involves all or part of the colon. It has periods of remission and exacerbation, and may even disappear for a while. The disease is slightly more common in women than in men. Onset of ulcerative colitis occurs between the ages of 15 and 50 in 75% of cases. (148) The incidence is lower in southern climates than in northern, and in blacks the incidence may be only one-third of whites. Incidence among Jews is three to five times greater than in non-Jews. (149)

In the United States between 200,000 and 400,000 have ulcerative colitis, and there are about 30,000 new cases diagnosed each year. (149)

Symptoms are diarrhea, abdominal pain of a cramping nature, rectal bleeding, weight loss, and weakness. Fever may be present. In one day the patient may pass 15 to 20 or more liquid stools which may contain blood, pus and mucus. (148) Malnutrition with weight loss and anemia are common. Abdominal tenderness is most common over the left colon, but may be present in any part of the abdomen. Only the rectum or rectosigmoid is involved in the early stages of the disease; as the disease progresses it advances up the colon. (148)

TREATMENT

1. Recently a sensitivity to cow's milk has been demonstrated in ulcerative colitis patients. (152) The person who suspects he might be developing ulcerative colitis should avoid all milk and foods containing milk (cheese, yogurt, sauces, gravies, and foods containing "whey" products, caseinates, lactates and milk solids). He must be very strict in his diet.

2. Babies should be breast-fed rather than bottle fed. (151) Babies have not yet developed a "mucosal barrier" to prevent milk antigens from attaching to the colon or getting into the blood stream. Most ulcerative colitis patients were given cow's milk as infants, not breast-fed.

3. Eggs, tomatoes, (154) beef, coffee, condiments, (155) spinach, and citrus fruits have all been implicated as factors contributing to ulcerative colitis and should be avoided on a trial basis.

4. Many patients improve significantly when placed on a gluten-free diet. All forms of wheat, rye, barley, oats, and buckwheat should be avoided. Labels of purchased foods should be scrutinized for any of these foods. As a general rule, millet and rice may be used freely. A trial on this diet for several weeks may prove to be quite rewarding.

5. Avoid very hot or very cold foods or liquids as these may irritate the gastrointestinal tract, or stimulate peristalsis and evacuation of the bowel, Irritants and stimulants such as coffee, tea, and other caffeine-containing beverages (chocolate, colas), alcohol, and carbonated beverages should be avoided.

6. Eat all foods, including soups and liquid foods, slowly. Chew thoroughly. Avoid overeating or compulsive eating.

7. Eat only two or three foods at a meal; the more food chemicals mixed, the greater the possibility of forming unfavorable compounds to cause a "war" in the stomach.

8. Eat only on a regular schedule. A two-meal a day schedule of the simplest foods will help the rest and recovery of the digestive system.

9. Some people find that eating carrots or carob will assist in controlling diarrhea. The pectin in bananas is felt to be helpful in diarrhea. (276)

10. Avoid the use of drugs of any type. A number of drugs can precipitate an exacerbation of ulcerative colitis, (153) and some cases of the disease have been traced to a course of oral antibiotics. Cortisone-type drugs, while producing temporary improvement in symptoms, do not favorably alter the course of the disease; however, complications related to corticosteroid therapy include osteoporosis, negative nitrogen balance, electrolyte imbalance, hypoglycemia, peptic ulcers, cataracts, pancreatitis, and a host of other disorders.

11. Because stress and emotional factors may produce a flare-up (153) we encourage out-of-doors exercise to tolerance, as exercise helps to neutralize stress.

12. Some people have to be taken off tap water and given only distilled water. Any of the chemicals in city water may cause a problem. Living in the country, and drinking well water would be ideal.

13. Hot enemas (115 to 122 degrees F.) may be used to stop bleeding. Such a temperature usually causes constriction of blood vessels. Lower temperatures (104 to 108 degrees F.) will discourage pain and increase circulation.

14. A cold sitz bath for 15 to 30 minutes with a hot foot bath may decrease diarrhea. Use a #2 wash tub from the hardware store for the cold water (about 92-94 degrees F.) and a foot tub for the hot water (108 to 112 degrees F.)

15. Hot sitz baths are beneficial to the circulation and the skin, and may be taken two or three times a day. During and after the bath, carefully protect the patient from chilling. (148)

16. An eight ounce glass of cabbage juice given before meals has been reported useful.

17. Bowel inflammation may be treated with a charcoal compress made with strong hops tea instead of water. Apply the compress at bedtime and leave it on all night. Drinking charcoal slurry water, three or four glasses a day, is often very helpful.

Make the slurry by stirring a tablespoonful of powdered charcoal into a glass of water; allow to settle, and drink the supernatant fluid.

18. Regularity in all things is essential. Have an established rising time, meal time, exercise time, and bed time. This schedule should apply seven days a week, 52 weeks a year, regardless of days off from work, holidays, etc. This enables the body to best utilize its natural circadian rhythms.

19. All animal products encourage putrefaction in the colon. Putrefaction by-products are irritating to the colon, and do not provide the most favorable bacterial flora.

20. A diet high in fiber, exercise, and a brief cold compress to the abdomen may be used to encourage proper bowel emptying. The high fiber diet should be introduced cautiously and gradually in a patient who has been on a low fiber diet for a long time.

21. Apply a compress for one to five minutes by wringing a large towel from ice water, and placing it over the abdomen.

22. A sugar-free, oil-free diet using only natural and unprocessed foods will assist the body in mobilizing its defense against infection.

23. Avoid vitamin and mineral supplements, and all other concentrated foods as these are stimulating, both to the bowel and the nervous system. Foods that have a high nutrient or caloric content per unit volume should be called "concentrated."

24. There are indications that ulcerative colitis may be viral in nature. A group of patients treated with artificial fever therapy, a treatment used successfully in some viral illnesses, all demonstrated improvement with a marked decrease in the number of stools per day, decreased rectal bleeding, and an increase in appetite with weight gain. The patients were given two and-a-half hours of treatment with rectal temperatures 104 to 105 degrees F., three times weekly, with an average of about 12 treatments per patient. (156)

25. Some herbal teas may be helpful: peppermint, goldenseal, and slippery elm bark have been recommended. Aloe vera may be soothing. Catnip tea will often quiet bowel action. A small goldenseal retention enema has been helpful.

26. Hot compresses to the abdomen with a simultaneous hot foot bath may be used for relief of pain.

27. Some very light exercise, such as walking, should be taken immediately after each meal to promote the quality of digestion.

28. Sunbaths can be taken daily to improve immune mechanisms and to encourage resistance to viral disease. Ulcerative colitis patients are unusually susceptible to infection.

29. Cooked brown rice or rice water will assist in the control of diarrhea. (312)

VAGINITIS

Vaginitis is an inflammation of the vagina. Most women experience it at some time during their lives. It may be caused by congestion of the pelvic organs, chemical irritation (strong douches), mechanical irritation (tampons), infection, and medications, especially antibiotics.

Symptoms of vaginitis are increased vaginal discharge, itching, vaginal pain or tenderness, painful intercourse, or painful urination.

There are three predominant types of vaginitis: yeast (Candida albicans), Trichomonas (Trichomonas vaginalis), and non-specific (caused by organisms other than those already mentioned).

Yeast vaginitis is also called monilial. It is more common in pregnant women, diabetics, and those on oral contraceptives, long-term steroid therapy or antibiotics.

Changes in the vaginal pH apparently allow the overgrowth of yeast. Tap water, tub baths and some preparations used in them, and some commercial douches may change the vaginal pH.

The discharge of yeast vaginitis is typically thick, yellowish or white, and curdlike. It is moderate in amount. There may be severe irritation of the external genital organs, causing much discomfort. (489)

Trichomonas vaginitis is caused by a protozoan, an organism which prefers a more alkaline area. It may be sexually transmitted from one partner to another and both should be treated at the same time. Symptoms in the female are a heavy yellow or greenish white, frothy discharge which may have a slight odor. The discharge is irritating, causing itching, burning, and redness of the skin. There may be frequency and burning with urination if the infection spreads to the urethra. Men are usually asymptomatic.

Flagyl has been given for this type of vaginitis in the past, but recent studies have shown that Flagyl causes cancer in animals.

Non-specific vaginitis may occur when host resistance is low and there is a change in the normal vaginal flora. There is profuse vaginal discharge with irritation of the external genitalia, and inflammation of the urethra.

TREATMENT

1. Yeast vaginitis may be treated by a hot soda water douche (1 to 3 teaspoons of soda to a quart of water) twice daily for seven days, then once daily for 30 days. If there is not prompt improvement it may be that the vaginitis is actually due to trichomonas and may be treated with a vinegar douche (1 to 4 tablespoons of vinegar to a quart of water) used on the same schedule as the soda water douche. A garlic water douche may be made by blending a single clove of garlic in part of a quart of boiling water. Add the remainder of the water and allow to stand until the temperature falls to about 110 degrees F. to denature the garlic enzyme. Use on the same schedule as the other douches. Warm normal saline (1 teaspoon salt per quart of water) has been reported useful in vaginitis caused by organisms other than trichomonas and Candida. (490)

2. Gentle cleansing of the perineum should be carried out front to back after every elimination. Cleaning from front to back prevents the possibility of contamination of the vaginal and urinary openings with fecal matter. (489)

3. Hot sitz baths taken two or three times per day may be soothing for local irritation. Clean the tub thoroughly before to prevent any possibility of introduction of bacteria from the tub to the vagina.

4. Sunshine, proper rest, and exercise, and good nutrition may be utilized to increase host resistance to organisms.

5. Avoid pantyhose, girdles, or synthetic pants or panties. Tight-fitting clothing encourages moisture retention, promoting growth of organisms. Cotton panties absorb moisture more readily than synthetic fabrics. (See section on cystitis.)

6. About 5% of women given tetracycline for acne develop vaginitis. (491)

7. Avoid the use of feminine hygiene sprays, or anything containing chemicals, tampons, and colored toilet tissues which are more likely to contain irritating substances.

8. Take showers instead of tub baths. Bath water may carry impurities into the vagina and urethra.

9. Wash undergarments carefully. Detergents sometimes remain in clothing and are irritating. Do not launder stockings, socks, and other footgear with under garments to avoid the possibility that yeast from the feet might be transferred to the vagina.

10. Use a low-fat, low-sugar diet to increase general resistance.

11. Avoid marital relations during infections. The partner should take a 20 minute sitz bath (110 degrees F.) twice daily for three days, then once daily for seven days, thoroughly cleansing the genitals with soap.

VARICOSE VEINS

A varicose vein is a vein in which the valves not longer function effectively, and which becomes stretched out of shape because of excess pressure. Varicose veins are one of the most common ailments of the circulatory system. Approximately 10% of the adult United States population have varicose veins sufficient to cause symptoms; 40 to 50% may have milder cases. (284)

The greater and lesser saphenous veins are the veins most often involved. When increased pressure is put on a deep vein the muscles surrounding it support it and keep it from getting out of shape. The saphenous veins, however, are located in the layer of fat just beneath the skin and do not receive muscle support.

Valves in the veins divide the veins up into individual chambers. When the veins do not function properly blood pools in the individual chambers, stretching them out of shape.

Symptoms of varicose veins are visibly distended veins. The skin may feel tense, ache or burn. There may be aching, a feeling of fullness in the limbs, or a sensation of tiredness. There may be muscle cramps, particularly at night. Discoloration of the skin, ranging from light brown to bluish, may be caused by hemorrhage under the skin.

Symptoms are often worse just prior to menstrual periods because of the vasodilation induced by hormones; contraceptive medicines may bring similar effects. (285)

Varicose veins are common during pregnancy. One study revealed that 62% of women first received medical attention for varicose veins after becoming pregnant. (283) The problem may subside after delivery of the infant, but recur, becoming worse with each subsequent pregnancy. Some women go through one or two pregnancies without problem only to have it occur with the next pregnancy. Varicose veins tend to be troublesome and enlarge rapidly during the first three months of pregnancy, then be less troublesome or even recede during the final three months.

Dr. Denis Burkitt, the well-known British researcher, believes that varicose veins, hemorrhoids, hiatus hernia, and colon diverticula are a result of increased abdominal pressures. The increased pressures come about by constipation and straining at the stool, which are consequences of our highly refined, fiber-depleted Western style diet. (535)

TREATMENT

1. Brisk walks for 15 minutes four times a day are beneficial for varicose veins. The blood is forced back toward the heart by the squeezing action of the calf muscles. (286)

2. Adequate dietary fiber is essential in the treatment of varicose veins. A full, distended colon applies pressure on the veins of the lower abdomen. This produces a slowing of the blood return to the heart, causing increased pressure in the leg veins.

3. Straining to move the bowels places pressure on the abominal veins, which in turn place pressure on the leg veins.

4. Knee-high stockings reduce blood flow, as do girdles, garter belts, and tight calf-high boots. No clothing should leave a mark on the skin. Avoid tight-fitting socks, shoes, or very high heeled shoes.

5. Hot baths or excessive sunbathing promote relaxation of the vein walls with accumulation of the blood, and may need to be avoided.

6. Sitting for long periods of time without walking around encourages stagnation of the venous blood. A brief walk every hour for only a minute is helpful during long sitting.

7. Swimming is an excellent exercise for patients with varicose veins. Swimming involves the lungs, heart, and legs and the pressure of the water on the leg veins serves as a pump.

8. Walking barefoot improves venous blood flow and exercises the muscles of the feet.

9. Crossing the legs at the knees restricts circulation and should be avoided.

10. Do not squat or sit back on your heels except for short periods during exercise.

11. Exercise your toes and rotate your ankles while standing or sitting.

12. Elastic stockings provide compression of the superficial veins, aiding upward movement of the blood. Put them on in the morning before getting out of bed. Pressure in the leg veins is five times greater in a standing position than when lying flat. Even tights provide a mild degree of compression (298) but severe cases of varicose veins require elastic stockings; even support hose are not adequate. Wear the stockings all the time except when in bed.

13. When weather prohibits walking, standing in place and rising up on the balls of the feet will tense the calf muscles. Repeat six to ten times frequently during the day.

14. Rest periods during the day with elevation of the legs will enlist the aid of gravity in returning blood to the heart.

15. During pregnancy, women may lift the weight of the baby off the vena cava and stimulate blood flow toward the heart by assuming a position on the knees and elbows. Place the palms, forearms, and elbows flat on the floor beneath the shoulders, knees should be directly under the hips. Keep the back straight; do not sag. You may raise the forearms off the floor, holding your head in the palms of your hands, for a slight change in position, or if you care to read.

16. If varicose veins become acutely painful lie down with legs elevated six inches higher than the heart. Apply warm compresses to the legs. Some people like to wring a towel out of hot water, and apply a hot water bottle over the towel to assist in keeping the compress warm.

17. Use a diet low in fats to prevent sluggish blood.

18. A shower twice a day may be very helpful, finishing off with a spray of cold water on the legs. (286) Using a hand shower attachment, massage one leg at a time, beginning with the toes and massaging upward toward the heart.

19. A light fingertip massage may be soothing to aching or swollen legs. Begin the massage at the toes, massage up toward the heart.

20. Raising the foot of the bed four to six inches will encourage return flow of the blood from the lower extremities to the heart.

21. Because of decreased blood flow patients with varicose veins sometimes develop skin ulcers. There are several treatments for them:

    A. Contrast baths are very helpful. For varicose veins uncomplicated by diabetes, immerse the foot up to the knee in a bucket of hot water at 104 degrees for two minutes, then in cold water for one minute, alternating back and forth for 20 minutes each day.

    B. Coat the ulcer with sterile petrolatum such as vaseline, then cover with gauze. Over the gauze place a three-quarter inch thick piece of sponge rubber large enough to extend over the ulcer margins about one inch on each side. Wrap a snug elastic bandage over all of it, extending the bandage about two inches above and below the ulcer. The dressing should be changed one to two times per week for a period of one to three weeks.

    C. Melt some plain gelatin in the top of a double boiler. Cover the ulcer with vaseline petroleum jelly or petrolatum. Cover this with sterile gauze. Wrap the leg from the bottom of the foot up to just below the knee with a layer of gauze, being careful not to fold or wrinkle it. Using about a two-inch paintbrush paint the warm liquid gelatin on the gauze. Wrap the leg with another layer of gauze, and paint as you did the first layer. Repeat the procedure four to five times and finish off with a heavy coat of gelatin. Leave this gelatin boot on for six days, continuing normal activities. Wash the leg with soap and water when the gelatin boot is removed, and apply rubbing alcohol. If the ulcer is not yet healed you may apply another boot in a day or two.

    D. Towels wrung out of warm, salty water and placed over the ulcer will stimulate healing. (288)

22. Sage washes and hot sage compresses may be useful, particularly for varicose ulcers. (309)

23. Deep breathing produces a strong negative pressure in the chest which pulls blood into the chest, decongesting the leg veins.

VENOUS THROMBOSIS

Venous thrombosis or blood clot in a vein, occurs in two forms, thrombophlebitis and phlebothrombosis. Thrombophlebitis denotes the presence of inflammation of the vein wall, whereas phlebothrombosis occurs with little or no inflammation.

Causes of venous thrombosis are injury to the blood vessel, blood stagnation or stasis, and increased clotting of the blood. Varicose veins, obesity, pregnancy, surgery, prolonged bed rest, lengthy automobile trips, and congestive heart failure may all cause venous stasis. Accelerated rates of clotting may be due to malignant neoplasms, blood abnormalities, oral contraceptives, dehydration, and a high fat or high protein diet.

Venous thrombi are made up mostly of red blood cells. The thrombus sticks to the vein wall but has a free-floating "tail;" it is this tail that often breaks free and travels to the lung. There is little hazard of embolism in frank thrombophlebitis, since the clot is usually densely adherent to the vessel wall; but there is great hazard in phlebothrombosis.

The increased incidence of venous thrombosis in women taking oral contraceptives is felt to be due to the effect of estrogens on the clotting mechanism.

Patients with venous thrombosis may have no or only mild symptoms. They may complain of an aching pain in the area at rest or during exercise. The pain is often worse on climbing hills or stairs if the calf is involved. With thrombophlebitis, the involved limb may swell, have elevated temperature, tenderness, distended veins, and a tender, firm cord felt in the tissues. Homan's sign, discomfort in the calf on upward flexion of the foot, is a nonspecific sign, but may be helpful in making the diagnosis. (520) Pain beneath an inflated blood pressure cuff over the involved area is an early sign of phlebitis.

Often the first sign of phlebothrombosis of a deep vein is a pulmonary embolism (clot in the lung).

PREVENTION AND TREATMENT

1. Deep breathing exercises produce increased negative pressure in the thorax, assisting in emptying large veins. (512) See Influenza for procedure. Persons in a high risk category as described above should often practice this exercise. Singing lustily offers similar protection.

2. Avoid dangling the feet, as pressure against the popliteal vessels may cause obstruction of blood flow.

3. Crossing the legs causes compression of blood vessels and should be avoided.

4. Eliminate the need to strain at stool by using adequate dietary fiber. Straining increases venous pressure in the legs.

5. Elevating the legs above the level of the heart utilizes gravity to return blood to the heart. Increased blood flow eliminates stasis and prevents formation of new thrombi. Venous pressure is also decreased by elevation of the legs, and relieves edema and pain. Placing the foot of the bed on six to eight inch high blocks is the best method of elevation. Using pillows under the legs frequently elevates the knee above the foot and interferes with blood flow. (513)

6. Avoid garters, girdles, and other tight clothing as these restrict blood flow.

7. Fasting decreases blood coagulation and may be beneficial. (514)

8. Regular exercise increases the body's ability to dissolve clots. (515)

9. A high-protein diet increases blood-clotting factors. (516)

10. Extended periods of sitting as when traveling, watching TV, etc., increase risk of venous stasis. Get up and walk about for a few minutes every hour.

11. Continuous applications of moist heat for 20 of every 24 hours are often recommended. They should cover the entire extremity. A simple method is to apply a thin layer of cold cream or petroleum jelly to the limb. Wring Turkish towels out of hot water and apply loosely. Cover them with a plastic or rubber cover. Use several hot water bottles or a waterproof electric heating pad set at "low" to maintain the heat. Cover the whole extremity with a dry blanket. The gentle heat will relieve venospasm and reduce discomfort. (517) Some people add 1 teaspoon of salt to each quart of water used to heat the towels.

12. Wading in water and swimming are excellent for preventing venous thrombosis. Water, denser than air, exerts an even pressure on the skin, assisting the return flow of venous blood.

13. Two minutes of exercise moving the legs as if riding the bicycle

every hour has been shown very effective in preventing thrombosis, particularly when combined with 15 rapid forced respira-
tions. (518)

14. Use a low fat diet and stay well hydrated to decrease blood
viscosity. Patients over 40 years of age with a hematocrit of 45%
or more have a 73% chance of developing deep vein thrombosis after surgery. (519)

15. For chronic, recurrent, disabling venous thrombosis, a novel
regimen of identification of food sensitivities and other environmental allergies has been described. The Texas researchers
reported complete control of a series of otherwise unrespon-
sive cases by using environmental control and avoidance of
offending foods. Comparison with a control group showed
striking benefits. (533)

16. The above listed treatments are for the most part indicated for
superficial venous thrombophlebitis. Phlebothrombosis of a
deep vein is a life-threatening event, and if suspected, should
be treated with hospitalization that would undoubtedly include anticoagulation and heparin, and possibly surgical pro-
cedures.

WARTS

Warts are caused by viruses. The tiny dark spots on the top of
warts are tiny hemorrhages or thrombosed capillaries.

Warts are slightly contagious. About 7% of school children have
warts. The peak incidence of warts is between 12 and 16 years,
then sharply declines.

The average wart disappears within a year. Ten to seventy five
percent of warts observed in one study over a short period of time
disappeared spontaneously.

TREATMENT

1. Apply several layers of waterproof adhesive tape to the wart,
and leave covered constantly for six-and-a-half days. With the
fingernail, scratch vigorously to remove all dead skin from the
wart possible. If the wart is still present, reapply the tape after
12 hours, and again leave on for six-and-a-half days. It may be
necessary to repeat this procedure several weeks. (362)

2. Comfrey poultices may be used. (363)

3. Sour apples contain magnesia. Some people report that paring the wart with a sharp razor blade and applying the juice of a sour apple works in the same manner as described in #1 above, as do also a few grains of epsom salts. (363)

4. The juice of white cabbage (363), aloe vera pulp, a tiny slice of garlic or raw potato, will each help remove warts if applied twice daily for several days to several weeks. Some warts respond quickly, some slowly.

5. Wheat germ oil may be applied to warts daily for two weeks.

6. Fifteen patients were instructed to soak their warts in hot water kept at 113 to 118 degrees F. for 30 to 90 minutes twice a week. Nine of the patients were cured. (369)

7. The milk of figs may be applied. One 15 year old girl had her wart disappear after only 3 applications. (367) Milkweed sap is also reported useful. Use one drop allowed to dry on the wart, applied daily for many days or even weeks.

8. One of the most simple treatments is to soak the wart in a concentrated salt water solution. To obtain a 30% solution add one and one-half teaspoon of salt to one-half cup of water. Soak the wart for 20 minutes two or three times a day for a few weeks. (368)

9. A small piece of cotton may be soaked in fresh pineapple juice, or a piece of crushed pulp attached to the wart. The enzymes in pineapple are said to dissolve a pared-down wart. (363)

10. Livia Warszawer-Schwarcz, M.D. of the Unit of Plastic Surgery at Rebacca Sieff Government Hospital in Safad, Israel, reports successful treatment of warts, particularly plantar warts, (the warts occurring on the sole of the foot) with a very simple procedure. The inner side of a fresh piece of banana skin is placed over the wart and held in place with tape. This is changed daily after washing the affected area. Once a week the thickened outer horny layer is removed. The maximum time required for the complete disappearance of the warts was six weeks and Dr. Warszawer-Schwarcz reported no recurrences in a two year follow up study. (364)

11. Two patients have been reported to develop multiple flat warts while receiving tetracycline. When the tetracycline was discontinued, the warts disappeared. (365) Other antibiotics may produce the same effects.

12. Sunlight has been shown helpful in the treatment of warts. Dr. W. E. Nelson, author of a prominent pediatrics textbook suggests sunlight exposure sufficient to cause redness of the skin. (366)

13. Castor oil may be applied to gauze and placed over the wart for half an hour three times a day.

APPENDIX A: COMMON FOOD ALLERGENS

1. Milk is the most common food allergen in the United States. Common sources of milk include whole, dried, skim, 2% and buttermilk, custards, cheese, cream and creamed foods, yogurt, sherbert, iced milk, and ice cream. Traces of milk are found in butter, breads, and many commercially prepared foods. Examine all foods for milk products such as lactose, milk solids, sodium caseinate, sodium lactate, milk fats and whey. Dr. Frederick Speer of the Speer Allergy Clinic says that all patients allergic to cow's milk are also allergic to goat's milk.

2. The kola nut family includes cola and chocolate. Both of these foods contain caffeine, as do coffee, tea, mate, cocoa and many soft drinks.

3. Corn is found in corn syrup, used in the manufacture of nearly all chewing gum, candy, prepared meats (luncheon meats, sausages, weiners, bologna), many baked goods, canned fruits, and fruit juices, jams, jellies, sweetened syrups, pancake syrups and ice cream. Hominy, grits, tortillas, Fritos, burritos, tamales, and enchiladas contain corn. Cornstarch is often used a thickener in soups and pies. Corn flour may be found in baked goods. Most American beer, bourbon, Canadian whiskey and corn whisky all contain corn. Corn oil should be avoided. Cornmeal is used in mush, scrapple, fish sticks, pancake, and waffle mixes.

4. Egg is capable of being such a potent allergen that even the odor of egg may produce symptoms. Many vaccines are egg-based. Baked goods, French toast, icings, meringue, candies, mayonnaise, salad dressings, meat loaves, breaded foods and noodles contain egg.

5. Legumes (the pea family) include peanut, soybean, and licorice. Mature ("dry") peas and beans are more likely to induce reactions than are green or string beans, or green peas. Many people sensitive to the legumes are also allergic to honey, probably because in the United States honey is gathered primarily from plants in the legume family. Soybean concentrates are common in baked goods, meats, and many manufactured foods. Soybean oil is the most commonly used oil in margarines, shortenings, salad oils, etc. Peanuts are able to produce severe reactions, including shock.

6. Citrus fruits including oranges, lemon, grapefruit, tangerine and lime are common allergens.

7. Tomato and apple are common in prepared foods. Apple is found in apple vinegar, pickles, salad dressings, etc. Tomato is found in meat loaf, soups, stews, pizza, catsup, chili, salads, tomato paste and juice, and many other prepared foods. Potato, eggplant, tobacco, red and bell pepper, cayenne, paprika, pimiento and chili pepper are all in the same family as tomato.

8. Wheat and small grains such as rice, barley, oats, rye, millet and wild rice may induce allergic reactions. This group also includes brown cane sugar, molasses, bamboo shoots, and sorghum. Wheat is the most allergenic, rye the least. Rye bread contains more wheat flour than rye flour. Buckwheat is a useful substitute for wheat.

   Wheat is found in many dietary products including all baked goods, gravies, cream sauces, macaroni, noodles, spaghetti, pie crusts, cereals, pretzels, chili and breaded foods.

9. Spices and food additives often induce allergic reactions. Cinnamon is found in catsup, candies, chewing gums, cookies, cakes, chili, prepared meats, apple dishes and pies. People who react to cinnamon usually react also to bay leaf. Pepper (black and white), cumin, basil, balm, hoarhound, marjoram, savory, rosemary, bergamot, coriander, sage, thyme, spearmint, peppermint, and oregano often cause reactions.

   Amaranth and tartrazine are possibly the artificial food colors most likely to produce symptoms. They are common in carbonated beverages, breakfast drinks such as Tang and Hi-C, bubble gum, popsicles, Kool-aid, Jello, and many medications.

10. Pork is the most common meat allergy, but oyster, clam, abalone, shrimp, crab, lobster, all true fish (such as tuna, salmon, catfish, and perch), chicken, turkey, duck, goose, pheasant, quail, beef, veal, lamb, rabbit, squirrel and venison may all induce symptoms.

After the elimination of offending foods some period of time may pass before the symptoms subside. Dr. Speer suggests that foods be eliminated for at least the following periods:

Milk	12 days
Wheat, rice, oats, barley	21 days
Corn	24 days
Egg	27 days
Tomato	30 days

Beans, peas, peanut   33 days
Citrus fruits   36 days
Apple   39 days

REFERENCES: Food Allergy: The 10 Common Offenders, American Family Physician 13(2):106-112, February 1976

Speer, Frederick, M.D. Allergy of the Nervous System, Springfield, Ill: C. C. Thomas, 1970

APPENDIX B: FOODS CONTAINING SALICYLATES

Potatoes
Cucumbers
Peppers
Tomatoes
Apples
Apricots
Blackberries
Boysenberries
Cherries
Currants
Dewberries
Gooseberries
Grapefruit

Lemons
Melons
Nectarines
Oranges
Peaches
Plums
Prunes
Raisins
Raspberries
Strawberries
Almonds
Grapes

REFERENCE: Archives of Dermatology 109:866, 1974

APPENDIX C: FAT FREE DIET

All foods contain fats and the needs of the average American are more than adequately met by these fats. Free fats, or fats added to foods may be restricted with great benefit to many people. We suggest the following guidelines:

1. Avoid the use of butter, margarine, salad dressings, mayonnaise, and nut butters such as peanut butter, etc. Use instead sauces made from blended fruits and vegetables.

2. Avoid fried foods and fatty snack foods such as French fries, potato chips, etc.

3. All meats contain excessive amounts of fat and should be avoided.

4. Milk and other dairy products, including cheese, are high in fat.

5. Eggs contain as much fat as they do protein.

APPENDIX D: LOW SALT DIET

Low salt means less than 800 to 1000 milligrams (about 1/2 tea-spoon) of salt per day. The average adult American eats 2,000 to 7,000 mg. of salt daily.

A few simple rules will enable anyone to have a low salt diet:

1. Do not add salt in cooking, or at the table.

2. Do not use commercially prepared foods such as bakery goods, etc. Canned vegetables usually contain salt. Fresh and frozen vegetables are generally satisfactory.

3. Many meats and all dairy products are high in sodium.

4. Use no foods containing baking soda, baking powder, mono-sodium glutamate, soy sauce, worcestershire sauce, catsup or mustard.

5. A number of medications including many antacids, Fleet's enema, Alka-seltzer, Metamucil, Effergel and others contain sodium.

APPENDIX E: PANCREAS RECOVERY DIET

1. Avoid all sugars including white, brown, and raw sugar, fructose, honey, syrups, jams, jellies, preserves, jello, etc.

2. Pies, cakes, sweetened desserts of any type, jello should not be used. Make your own healthful desserts without sugar. A cookbook such as *EAT FOR STRENGTH* will be helpful.

3. Cheese and milk and milk products are best eliminated. Milk contains leucine which has been shown to induce hypoglycemic syndrome.

4. Refined grains including white breads, crackers, saltines, white macaroni, white rice, spaghetti, and other refined grain foods should be replaced with whole grain products.

5. Extremely sweet fruits such as raisins, dates, figs, etc., are concentrated foods and are best eliminated for at least a year after beginning the diet. After a year small amounts may be introduced on a trial basis, and used if no symptoms develop. Bananas, watermelon, mangoes and sweet potatoes are all in this category. Grapes may induce symptoms in some people.

6. Caffeine, nicotine, and alcohol are all harmful to the blood sugar regulating mechanisms of the body. Coffee, tea, cola drinks, and chocolate all contain caffeine. Many over-the-counter medications contain caffeine.

7. All soft drinks contain excessive amounts of sugars or sweeteners. This includes Kool-aid. Fruit juices are concentrated foods and should be used sparingly if at all. It is much better to use the whole fruit.

8. Spices have an adverse effect on the nervous system and may aggravate symptoms. Vinegar and vinegar-containing foods may be prepared using lemon juice and salt in place of the vinegar.

APPENDIX F: DIGESTION

The interdigestive phase of bowel activity is a special cleansing phase. Diseases such as inflammations, ulcerations, and other malfunctions are more likely to afflict the intestinal tract if the bowel fails to get this cleansing phase after each meal.

The intestinal tract cannot enter this phase of activity unless the stomach and small bowel are free of all food and food residues. Immediately upon completion of moving all food residues from the stomach and small bowel into the colon, the upper gastrointestinal tract slips into the interdigestive phase. This phase is characterized by a different pace and length of activity, with a difference in the size of the segment of the intestinal tract involved with a peristaltic wave. The secretion of the bowel is different as are fluid shifts across membrane surfaces.

Many individuals never experience an interdigestive phase, as they never have an empty stomach and small bowel. Eating between meals and at irregular meal times forces the bowel to always maintain the digestive phases, and to be deprived of the essential cleaning activity of the interdigestive phase. A usual meal requires about four hours to clear the upper intestinal tract providing nothing is eaten between meals. Eating or drinking nourishing beverages between meals delays emptying by several hours. Eating at bedtime almost insures that some food will be in the intestinal tract during the night and into the next day.

BIBLIOGRAPHY

1. Beeson, Paul, M.D., Walsh McDermott, M.D. and James F. Wyngaarden, M.D. Cecil Textbook of Medicine, 15th Edition, Phil: W. B. Saunders, 1979, pp. 1223-1229
2. Isselbacher, Kurt J., M.D. Harrison's Principles of Internal Medicine. New York: McGraw-Hill, 1980, pp. 1118-1119
3. Hurst, J. Willis. The Heart. Fifth Edition. New York: McGraw-Hill, 1982. pp. 1021-1024
4. Annals of Internal Medicine 69:529-536, September, 1968
5. Journal of the American Medical Association 158(12):1008-1013, July 23, 1955
6. The Lancet 1:1325-1327, June 12, 1982
7. American Heart Journal 93(6):803-804, June, 1977
8. Behrman, Howard T., Theodore A. Labow, M.D. and Jack H. Rozen, M.D. Common Skin Diseases. New York: Grune and Stratton, 1978. p. 9
9. Luckmann, Joan, R.N. and Karen Sorensen, R.N. Medical Surgical Nursing: A Psychophysiologic Approach. Philadelphia: W. B. Saunders Company. 1980
10. Wyngaarden, James B., M.D. and Lloyd Smith Jr., M.D. Cecil Textbook of Medicine, 16th Edition, Philadelphia: W. B. Saunders, 1982, pp. 618-619
11. Phipps, Wilma J., R.N., Barbara C. Long, R.N. and Nancy Woods, R.N. Shafers Medical Surgical Nursing. St. Louis: C. V. Mosby Company. 1980. p. 586
12. Annals of Allergy 44:302-307, May, 1980
13. Consultant, July, 1976, p. 103, 105
14. Hoekelman, Robert A. et al. Principles of Pediatrics. New York: McGraw-Hill, 1978 p. 1790
15. Whalley, Lucille, R.N. and Donna L. Wong, R.N. Nursing Care of Infants and Children. St. Louis: C. V. Mosby, 1979, p. 309
16. Brunner, Lilliam R.N. and Doris Suddarth, R.N. The Lippincott Manual of Nursing Practice. Philadelphia: Lippincott, 1982 p. 1354
17. A.M.A. Journal of Diseases of Children 94:234, 1957
18. Cooke, Robert E., M.D. and Sidney Levin, M.D. The Biologic Basis of Pediatric Practice. New York: McGraw Hill 1968 p. 223
19. Rudolph, Abraham M.D. Pediatrics. 16th Edition. New York: Appleton-Century-Crofts, 1977 p. 927-928
20. Clinical Pediatrics 14(2)129, February, 1975
21. Hoekelman, op. cit. page 1790

22. Shirkey, Harry C. Pediatric Therapy. 6th Edition. St. Louis: C. V. Mosby, 1980, p. 541
23. British Veterinary Journal 136:448, 1980
24. Brunner. op. cit. p. 584
25. Phipps, op. cit. p. 870
26. Contact Dermatitis 6(4):287, June 1980
27. New England Journal of Medicine 303(10)583 Sept. 4, 1980
28. Journal of the American Medical Association 39:441, 1902
29. Surgical Clinics of North America 58(3)505-512, June, 1978
30. Southern Medical Journal 61:1005-1006, 1968
31. Wyngaarden, op. cit. p. 747-748
32. Ohio State Medical Journal 70:425-6, July, 1974
33. Diseases of the Colon and Rectum 20(1)40-42, January-February, 1977
34. Moschella, Samuel L., M.D., Donald M. Pillsbury, M.D. and Harry J. Hurley, Jr., M.D. Dermatology, Volume 1. Philadelphia: W. B. Saunders Company, 1975. pp. 639-644
35. Tierra, Michael. The Way of Herbs. Santa Cruz, CA: Unity Press, 1980 p. 73
36. Brunner. op cit. p. 579
37. Journal of the American Medical Association 130:249-256, 1946
38. Graedon, Joe. The People's Pharmacy. New York: St. Martin's Press, 1976 p. 105
39. The Medical Letter on Drugs and Therapeutics 18(4)17-18, February 13, 1976
40. British Medical Journal 4:758, December 26, 1970
41. Canadian Medical Association Journal 71:492 November, 1954
42. Archives of Internal Medicine 115:155-159, February, 1965
43. Journal of Clinical Psychiatry 39(9):693-8, September, 1978
44. Acta Medica Scandinavica 164:231-232, 1959
45. Williams, Sue Rodwell, Ph.D. Nutrition and Diet Therapy. St. Louis: C. V. Mosby Co. 1977
46. Davidson, Sr. Stanley, Reg Passmore, John F. Brock and A. Stewart Truswell. Human Nutrition and Dietetics. New York: Churchill Livingstone, 1979
47. Journal of Applied Nutrition 26(4):8-15, Fall, 1974
48. Munchener Medizinische Wochenschrift, Oct. 5, 1909
49. University Hospital Bulletin, June, 1935 p. 19
50. American Practitioner, July, 1948, p. 708
51. Journal of Allergy 27:382-3, 1956
52. Journal of the American Medical Association 169:1158, March 14, 1959

53. British Medical Journal 1:669, March 18, 1978
54. American Review of Respiratory Disease 84:480, 1961
55. Medical Journal of Australia 1:608, April 24, 1976
56. Journal of Allergy 45:310-319, May, 1970
57. Medical Journal of Australia 2:614-617, Nov. 28, 1981
58. Life and Health, June, 1909, p. 375
59. Guyton, Arthur, M.D. Basic Human Physiology. Philadelphia: W. B. Saunders, 1977, p. 82
60. Annals of Allergy 42:160-165, March, 1979
61. Brunner. op cit. p. 622
62. The Health Letter, September 24, 1976, p. 1-4
63. Graedon. op. cit. p. 178
64. Ibid. p. 176-177
65. Journal of the American Medical Association 231:1017-1018, 1975
66. Pediatrics 45:150-151, January, 1970
67. Science News Letter 85:374, June 13, 1964
68. Medical Journal of Australia 1:612, April 24, 1976
69. Medical Self-Care, Summer, 1981, pp. 44-47
70. Pediatric Clinics of North America 16(1): 31-42, February, 1969
71. Arzneimittel-Forsch 6:445-450, 1956
72. American Journal of Public Health 72:574-579, 1982
73. Science News, February 16, 1935 p. 105
74. Clinical Allergy 11(6)549-553, 1981
75. Helvetica Medica Acta 20:433-433, November, 1953
76. American Practitioner 3:551, May, 1948
77. Vaughan, Victor C. M.D. et al. Nelson Textbook of Pediatrics. Philadelphia: W. B. Saunders Co. 1979, p. 208-209
78. Rudolph. op. cit. p. 1011
79. The Lancet 2:437-439, August 26, 1978
80. The Lancet 2:261, August 1, 1981
81. The Lancet 2:734, September 30, 1978
82. McMillan, Julia A. M.D., Phillip Inieburg, M.D. and Frank Oski, M.D. The Whole Pediatricians Catalog. Philadelphia: Saunders. 1977.
83. Archives of Pediatrics 38:756, 1921
84. American Journal of Diseases of Children 133:996, October, 1979
85. Crook, William G. M.D. Answering Parents Questions. Springfield: C. C. Thomas, 1963
86. Archives of Pediatrics 75(7)271-278, July, 1958
87. American Journal of Roentology 38:779-780, November, 1937
88. The Lancet 1:1340-1342, June 20, 1981

89. Medical Journal of Australia 1(10)542, May 16, 1981
90. Pediatrics 69:117-118, January, 1982
91. Whalley. op. cit. p. 494
92. New York Journal of Medicine 57:265, Jan. 15, 1957
93. Annals of Allergy 29:323-324, June, 1971
94. British Medical Journal 1(3147)601, April 23, 1971
95. McFarlane, Judith M., R.N. et al. Contemporary Pediatric Nursing: A Conceptual Approach. New York: Wiley, 1980 p. 120
96. Whalley. op. cit. p. 492-493
97. Luckmann. op cit. p. 955-956
98. Medical Self Care, Spring, 1981, p. 9-14
99. Kilmartin, Angela. Cystitis: The Complete Self-Help Guide. Warner Books, 1980
100. Annals of Internal Medicine 1:117-126, Sept. 1972
101. Luckmann. op. cit. p. 1873-1875
102. Journal of the American Medical Association 62:1297-1301, April 25, 1914
103. Moor, Fred, M.D. et al. Manual of Hydrotherapy and Massage. Mountain View, Ca. Pacific Press Publishing Association, 1964 p. 42, 45
104. Archives of Surgery 46:611-613, May, 1943
105. Journal of the Association for Physical and Mental Rehabilitation 18:97-109, July-August, 1964
106. Journal of the Mississippi Medical Association 28:382, 1931
107. Journal of Obstetrics and Gynecology of the British Commonwealth 42:309-317, 1935
108. Budoff, Penny M.D. No More Menstrual Cramps and Other Good News. New York: G. P. Putnam Sons, 1980
109. Journal of Reproductive Medicine 25(4 Suppl):198-201, October, 1980
110. Gerrard, John, Food Allergy. Springfield: C. C. Thomas, 1980 p. 169-185
111. Canadian Medical Association Journal 106:30, 1972
112. Clinical Trends in Family Practice. Sept.-October, 1978
113. GP 20:84-98, December, 1959
114. Modern Medicine, September 30, 1977 p. 43
115. Rocky Mountain Medical Journal 57:50-2, June 1960
116. Medical Tribune, April 9, 1980 p. 20
117. Brunner. op cit. p. 132-133
118. Patient Care, February 15, 1978 p. 183
119. Life and Health, February, 1914, p. 89

120. Journal of the American Medical Association 150:760-764, October 25, 1952
121. British Medical Journal 1:1233, May 4, 1963
122. Journal of the American Medical Association 202(3)173-174, October 16, 1967
123. Presse Medica 36:1020, August 11, 1928
124. Journal of the American Medical Association 196(1):226, April 4, 1966
125. Family Practice News, April 1, 1978
126. Ear, Nose and Throat Journal 58:354-357, August, 1979
127. Clark, Ann L. Childbearing: A Nursing Perspective. Philadelphia: F.A. Davis, 1979 p. 739
128. Lerch, Constance, R.N. and Jane Bliss, R.N. Maternity Nursing. St. Louis: C. V. Mosby, 1978, p. 372-373
129. Bleier, Inge J., R.N. Maternity Nursing: A Textbook for Practical Nurses. Philadelphia W. B. Saunders, 1971, p. 193
130. Reeder, Sharon, R.N., Ph.D., Maternity Nursing. 14th Edition. Philadelphia: J. B. Lippincott, 1980 p. 486
131. Bookmiller, Mae M., R.N. et al. Textbook of Obstetrics and Obstetrics Nursing. Philadephia: W. B. Saunders, 1967 p. 449-450
132. Bryant, Richard, M.D. and Anna E. Overland, R.N. Woodward's and Gardner's Obstetric Management and Nursing. Philadelphia: F. A. Davis, 1964 p. 132
133. Child-Family Digest 19:45, 1960
134. Canadian Nurse 72(3):32, March, 1976
135. Abbott, George, M.D., Fred Moor, M.D. and Kathryn Jensen-Nelson, R.N. Physical Therapy in Nursing Care. Takoma Park, Washington, D.C. Review and Herald Publishing Association. 1945 p. 350
136. Clinical Obstetrics and Gynecology 5(1)59-60, March, 1962
137. Postgraduate Medicine 30:47-50, July, 1961
138. Journal of the American Medical Association 244(20)2332-2333, November 21, 1980
139. Journal of the American Medical Association 246(7):732, August 14, 1981
140. The New England Journal of Medicine 301:216 July 26, 1979
141. Brunner. op. cit. p. 996
142. Physiotherapy 45:169, July-August, 1959
143. American Practitioner 11:799-806, September, 1960
144. Consultant, March, 1981, p. 20
145. Medical Times, May, 1978 p. 3

146. The Lancet 1:202-203, January 27, 1973
147. California Medicine 92:204-206, March, 1960
148. Phipps. op. cit. p. 604-605
149. Wyngaarden, op cit. p. 703-711
150. Voprosy Pitaniia 17(3):55-61, 1958
151. British Medical Journal (5257):929-933, October 7, 1961
152. Archives of Internal Medicine 113:519-522, April, 1964
153. Goodman, Michael J and Marshall Sparberg. Ulcerative Colitis. New York: John Wiley, 1978, p. 134-137
154. Goodhart, Robert and Maurice Shills, Modern Nutrition in Health and Disease. New York: Lea and Febiger, 1980 p. 940
155. American Journal of Gastroenterology 34:49-66, July, 1960
156. Journal of the American Medical Association 109:2017, December 11, 1937
157. American Journal of Nursing 81:1007-1009, May, 1981
158. Wyngaarden. op cit. p. 322-323
159. Seminars in Arthritis and Rheumatism 10(4) 282-302, 1981
160. Medical Journal of Australia 2:371, September 7, 1974
161. New England Journal of Medicine 303(24) 1419, December 11, 1980
162. American Heart Journal 74:229-234, 1967
163. The Lancet 288:1086-1088, May 22, 1965
164. Archives of Surgery 110:1343-1346, November 1975
165. Physical Therapeutics 47:215-225, April, 1929
166. Journal of the American Medical Association 240(25):2760, December 15, 1978
167. Journal of the American Medical Association 242(26)2845, December 28, 1979
168. Executive Health 10(2):1-4, 1973
169. Science News 119(1):3, January 3, 1981
170. Journal of the American Medical Association 53:1242, 1909
171. Patient Care, March 15, 1973 p. 86
172. Klinische Wochenschrift 15:1885-1886, 1936
173. New England Journal of Medicine 295(5):260-262, July 29, 1976
174. American Journal of Digestive Diseases 17:383-389, May, 1972
175. Medical Clinics of North America 62(1):155-164, January, 1978
176. Postgraduate Medicine 57(1):77-80, January, 1975
177. Beeson. op. cit. p. 1489
178. Bockus, Henry L. et al. Gastroenterology, Third Edition, Volume 4. Philadelphia: W. B. Saunders, 1976, p. 660-663
179. Science News 118(19):301, November 8, 1980
180. New England Journal of Medicine 302(26) 1474-1475, June 26, 1980

181. Internal Medicine News 10(19):23, October 1, 1977
182. Review of Gastroenterology 11:22-26, Jan-Feb. 1944
183. Review of Gastroenterology 16:411-419, May, 1949
184. Brunner. op cit. p. 398-401
185. Wyngaarden. op cit. p. 635-640
186. Phipps. op cit. p. 594-600
187. Family Practice News, June 15, 1978
188. Circulation 21:538-42, April, 1960
189. Current Prescribing, May, 1977 p. 93
190. Hospital Practice, July, 1976 p. 33-38
191. Internal Medicine News 13(13):1, 21
192. New England Journal of Medicine 282:1402-1405, June 18, 1970
193. Journal of the American Medical Association 244(22):2544-2546, December 5, 1980
194. Gastroenterology 76:603-606, March, 1979
195. Annals of Internal Medicine 82:546, April, 1975
196. Modern Medicine 48(2):123-124, Feb. 15, 1980
197. Postgraduate Medicine 63(4):83, April, 1978
198. Hospital Medicine 15(8)47-59, August, 1979
199. Journal of the American Medical Association 126(13)819, November 25, 1944
200. Science News 93:451, May 11, 1968
201. Journal of the American Medical Association 241(5)439, February 2, 1979
202. Journal of the American Dietetic Association 26:668-672, September, 1950
203. California Medicine 70:10-15, January, 1949
204. Journal of the American Osteopathic Association 62:731-735, April, 1963
205. British Medical Journal, February 16, 1980, p. 483-484
206. Gut 18:725-729, September, 1977
207. Newsweek, October 29, 1956
208. Medical Journal of Australia 1:7-8, Jan. 2, 1943
209. Gastroenterologia 91:315-326, 1959
210. Hospital Practice 14:55, December, 1979
211. American Heart Journal 98(5):666-668, Nov. 1979
212. Physiotherapy 66(8)260-261, August, 1980
213. Angiology 22(1)1-3, January, 1971
214. Biorheology 13:161-164, 1976
215. Journal of the American Medical Association 95(25)1910-1911, December 20, 1930
216. Wyngaarden. op cit. p. 1107-1118

217. Davidson. op. cit. p. 437-443
218. Howard, Rosanne and Nancie Herbold. Nutrition in Clinical Care. New York: McGraw-Hill 1978, p. 439-441
219. Parade, July 4, 1982 p. 16
220. Internal Medicine News July 15, 1980
221. Scottish Medical Journal 18:Suppl:239-242, 1973
222. Nature 228:180, October 10, 1970
223. British Journal of Physical Medicine 6:250-251, March, 1932
224. Texas Report on Biology and Medicine 8:309-311, 1950
225. Journal of the American Dietetic Association 29:441-442, 1953
226. The Lancet 2:67-68, July 12, 1952
227. New Zealand Medical Journal 85:349, April 27, 1977
228. Geriatrics 35(5):69-78, May, 1980
229. Davidson. op. cit. p. 438
230. Beeson. op. cit. p. 731-732
231. Pryse-Phillips, William, M.D. and T. J. Murray. Essential Neurology. Garden City, New York: Medical Examination Pub. Co. 1978 p. 227
232. Archives of Neurology 36(12)784-790, Nov. 16, 1979
233. Journal of the American Medical Association 239(22):2380-2383, June 2, 1978
234. Postgraduate Medicine 56(659)617-621, Sept. 1980
235. Wyngaarden. op. cit. p. 1949-1951
236. Hills, Hilda Cherry. Good Food to Fight Migraine. New Canaan, Ct: Keats Publishing Co. 1981
237. Journal of Human Nutrition 34:175-180, 1980
238. Internal Medicine News 10(2):15, Jan. 15, 1977
239. The Lancet 1(8123):966-9, May 5, 1979
240. The Lancet 2(7245):53, July 7, 1962
241. Archives of Otolaryngology 75:220, 1962
242. The Lancet 2(8184)1-3, July 5, 1980
243. Minnesota Medicine 59(4):232-3, April, 1976
244. Medical World News, July 12, 1968, p. 25
245. Modern Medicine, February 8, 1971, p. 100-6
246. Journal of the American Medical Association 222(6)703, November 6, 1972
247. British Medical Journal 284:312, Jan. 30, 1982
248. The Physician and Sportsmedicine 9(8):24-25, August, 1981
249. Family Practice News, May 1, 1980, p. 40
250. Headache 20(1)42-43, January, 1980
251. Journal of the American Medical Association 239(23):2481, June 9, 1978

252. Wyngaarden. op. cit. p. 1963
253. Phipps. op. cit. p. 320-321
254. Annals of Otology, Rhinology and Laryngology, July-August, 1975
255. Medical World News, October 22, 1971, p. 34E
256. Brunner. op. cit. p. 698
257. Ear, Nose, and Throat Journal 56(4):160-3, April, 1977
258. Luckmann. op cit. p. 1705-1711
259. The Palm Beach Post, February 10, 1982 p. A-8
260. SIP Newsletter, January 11, 1980
261. American Family Physician, 23:237-241, February, 1981
262. The Lancet 1(8273):623, March 13, 1982
263. International Archives of Allergy and Applied Immunology 64:287-292, 1981
264. Acta Medica Scandinavica 192:231-239, 1972
265. Arthritis and Rheumatism 17(3)229, May-June 1974
266. Acta Rheumatologica Scandinavica 11:161-168, 1965
267. Proceedings of the Royal Society of Medicine 30:1-10, 1936
268. Canadian Nurse 56(4):325, April, 1960
269. Consultant, July 1981, p. 171-175
270. The Lancet 2:1550, December 10, 1938
271. RN, September, 1982 p. 137
272. Homola, Samuel, D.C. Doctor Homola's Natural Health Remedies. West Nyack, NY: Parker Publishing Co. 1973 p. 230
273. Ibid, p. 43
274. Ibid. p. 134
275. Ibid. p. 150
276. Ibid. p. 156
277. Wyngaarden. op. cit. p. 319
278. Phipps. op. cit. p. 1031-1032
279. Brunner. op. cit. p. 348
280. Phipps. op. cit. p. 1020-1021
281. Brunner. op. cit. p. 333-334
282. Basmajian, John V. Therapeutic Exercise, Third Edition, Baltimore: Williams and Wilkins, 1978, p. 533-534
283. Baron, Howard C. M.D. Varicose Veins: A Commonsense Approach To Their Management. New York: William Morrow, 1979
284. Postgraduate Medicine 65(6):131, June, 1979
285. Postgraduate Medicine 65(6):132, June, 1979
286. Medical Tribune 26(8):2, February 27, 1980
287. British Medical Journal 1:254, Jan. 31, 1976

288. Homola. op. cit. p. 32-33
289. Canadian Medical Association Journal 126:1281-1285, June 1, 1982
290. New York State Journal of Medicine 34:282-289, 1934
291. Journal of the American Dental Association 55:37-46, July, 1957
292. The New York Journal of Dentistry 12(5)192-197, May, 1942
293. Buchman, Dian Dincin. Herbal Medicine, New York: Gramercy Publishing Co. 1979, p. 91
294. Ibid. p. 173
295. Ibid. p. 172-173
296. Ibid. p. 8
297. Ibid. p. 9
298. Ibid. p. 60
299. Ibid. p. 143
300. Ibid. p. 155
301. Ibid. p. 60
302. Ibid. p. 75
303. Ibid. p. 77
304. Ibid. p. 77
305. Ibid. p. 145
306. Ibid. p. 60
307. Ibid. p. 77
308. Ibid. p. 167
309. Ibid. p. 109
310. Ibid. p. 140
311. Ibid. p. 171
312. Ibid. p. 143
313. American Family Physician 4(4)75-76, Oct. 1971
314. Rook, Arthur et al. Textbook of Dermatology Volume 1. New York: Blackwell, 1979, p. 549-551
315. Domonkos, Anthony et al. Andrew's Diseases of the Skin. Philadelphia: Saunders, 1982 p. 275-277
316. Medical Times 107(2):34d-39d, Feb. 1979
317. Phipps. op. cit. p. 556-557
318. Family Practice News 9(12):35, June 15, 1979
319. Internal Medicine News 12(16)1, 16, Sept. 1, 1979
320. Medical World News, July 6, 1981, p. 46, 48
321. Gastroenterology 82:822, 1982
322. Family Practice News, Sept. 1, 1978 p. 2
323. British Medical Journal 1:1265, May 12, 1979
324. Journal of the American Medical Association 122:444, June 12, 1943

325. The Lancet 2:1198-1199, November 27, 1971
326. American Journal of Gastroenterology 25:158-163, February, 1956
327. Science News Letter 86:263, Oct. 24, 1964
328. Annals of Allergy 26:83-89, 1968
329. Breneman, J. C. M.D. Basics of Food Allergy. Springfield: C. C. Thomas, 1978, p. 68
330. American Journal of Surgery 135:321, March, 1978
331. Internal Medicine News 11(9):18, May 1, 1978
332. American Journal of Digestive Diseases 14:531-537, 1969
333. Medical Tribune, August 23, 1978
334. American Family Physician, 18:171 October, 1978
335. American Journal of Clinical Nutrition 32:2174-2176, November, 1979
336. Thompson, W., Irritable Gut. University Park, 1978 p. 65-84
337. Isselbacher, Kurt J. M.D. et al. Harrison's Principles of Internal Medicine, New York: McGraw-Hill, 1980 p. 1422-1423
338. Drug Therapy, August 1982, p. 61-64
339. American Family Physician 11(3):168-173, March, 1975
340. Wyngaarden, pp. 669-670
341. Consultant, June 1981, p. 25-29
342. Sleisenger, Marvin H. and Fordtran, John Gastrointestinal Disease. Philadelphia: Saunders, 1978, p. 1585-1597
343. Bargen, J. Arnold. The Modern Management of Colitis. Springfield: C. C. Thomas, 1943, p. 39
344. Medical Clinics of North America 61(1):207, January, 1978
345. Modern Medicine, July 15, 1977, p. 36-40
346. Hospital Medicine, May, 1981, pp. 36A-36J
347. Drug Therapy, August, 1982, p. 46
348. Postgraduate Medicine, October, 1980, p. 64
349. The Lancet 2:417-418, August 27, 1977
350. The Lancet 1:540, March 6, 1976
351. American Journal of Clinical Nutrition 27:106, February, 1974
352. Walker-Smith, John M.D. Diseases of the Small Intestine in Childhood. 2nd Edition, Pitman Medical, 1979, pp. 91-138
353. Nursing Times 69:1213-1215, Sept. 20, 1973
354. Lorenzen, Evelyn J., Ph.D., M.D. Editor. Dietary Guidelines. Houston: Gulf Pub. Co. 1978, p. 71-76
355. Nursing Times 71(2):806-808, May 22, 1975
356. Shirkey, Harry C. Pediatric Therapy. 6th Edition St. Louis: C.V. Mosby Co. 1980, p. 610-613
357. Clinics in Gastroenterology 3:149-211, Jan. 1974
358. Nursing Times 73(44)1708-1710, Nov. 3, 1977

359. Archiv fur Kinderheilkunde 102:106-116, 1934
360. American Journal of Diseases of Children 28:421, October, 1924
361. British Medical Journal 1:152, Jan. 18, 1975
362. Hospital Medicine, November, 1980, p. 47
363. Buchman. op. cit.
364. Plastic and Reconstructive Surgery 68(6) 975-976, December, 1981
365. Archives of Dermatology 111:930, July, 1975
366. Nelson, Waldo E. Mitchell-Nelson Textbook of Pediatrics. Philadelphia: W. B. Saunders Company, 1954, pp. 1560-1561
367. South African Medical Journal 56(6)205, August 11, 1979
368. Graedon. op. cit. p. 100
369. Cleveland Clinic Quarterly 29:156, 1962
370. American Family Physician 8(6):100-107, December, 1973
371. Luckmann. op. cit. pp. 2055-2058
372. Journal of the American Medical Association 111:1744-1746, November 5, 1938
373. Phipps. op. cit. p. 331-332
374. Buchman. op. cit. p. 75, 174
375. Levine, Howard L. M.D. Diagnosis and Management of Sinusitis. #2012 Southern Medical Association Dial Access. 1979
376. Homola. op. cit. p. 48-49
377. Today's Clinician, April, 1978 p. 43-45
378. Consultant, July, 1976, pp. 27-29
379. Phipps. op. cit. p. 607-608
380. The Lancet 1:664-666, 1977
381. Patient Care, January 30, 1979, p. 167
382. Internal Medicine News, February 1, 1975, p. 3
383. Archives of Pathology 36:621, December, 1943
384. Modern Medicine, October 15-30, 1980, pp. 41-48
385. British Medical Journal 1:929, April 6, 1963
386. British Medical Journal 1:1290, May 11, 1963
387. Nurse-Practitioner November-December, 1976, p. 13-16
388. Phipps. op. cit. p. 823-824
389. New England Journal of Medicine 267(6)297-299, August 9, 1962
390. Journal of the American Medical Association 162(11)1041-1043, November 14, 1956
391. American Family Physician 23(6):186, June, 1981
392. Medical Record, August 26, 1916, p. 367-8

393. Journal of Neural Transmission 51:135-148, 1981
394. Wyngaarden, op. cit. p. 2025-2029
395. Williams, Paul C. Back and Neck Pain. Springfield: C. C. Thomas, 1974, pp. 36-42
396. American Family Physician 10(4)190, October, 1974
397. Journal of the American Medical Association 242(26)2845, December 28, 1979
398. Archives of Physical Medicine and Rehabilitation 62:96, February, 1981
399. Medical World News, March 1, 1982 p. 29
400. National Enquirer, October 17, 1979
401. Consultant, November, 1980, p. 29
402. JOGN Nursing 11(2)103-107, March-April, 1982
403. Annals of Internal Medicine 89:356-358, 1978
404. Clinics in Endocrinology 2(2)180, July, 1973
405. Wyngaarden. op. cit. pp. 1331-1336
406. Family Practice News, August 1, 1978, p. 8
407. New England Journal of Medicine 273:73, 1965
408. Journal of Nutrition 46:181, 1952
409. The Lancet 2:423, August 21, 1982
410. Journal of Gerontology 4:185-192, July, 1949
411. Proceedings of the Nutrition Society 38(2)61A, September, 1979
412. American Journal of Clinical Nutrition 14:98, 1964
413. Columbus Ledger, June 16, 1982
414. Journal of the American Medical Association 247(8)1106-1107, February 26, 1982
415. Journal of the American Medical Association 221:509, 1972
416. Medical Tribune, March 14, 1973 p. 3
417. Biological Sciences, April 28, 1973
418. Geriatrics 36(9)71-79, September, 1981
419. Hospital Tribune, July 28, 1969
420. Medical World News, February 21, 1969, p. 18-19
421. Archives of Oral Biology 26:393-397, 1981
422. Phipps. op. cit. p. 531-532
423. Internal Medicine News, April 1, 1979 p. 37 November-December, 1957
425. British Journal of Radiology 34:429, 1961
426. Journal of the American Medical Association 198(5)85, October 31, 1966
427. Medical Opinion, January, 1977 p. 14-22

428. Goodhart, Robert M.D. and Shils, Maurice M.D. Modern Nutrition in Health and Disease Philadelphia: Lea and Febiger, 1980 p. 870
429. Wohl, Michael and Goodhart, Robert S. Modern Nutrition in Health and Disease. 4th Edition p. 142
430. Osteoporosis. Marion Laboratories, Inc. No date. p. 2
431. American Journal of Anthropology 44(1)111-112, January, 1976
432. Ballentine, Rudolph, M.D. Diet and Nutrition, Himalayan Press, 1978
433. Wyngaarden. op. cit. p. 711-719
434. Phipps. op. cit. p. 1286-1287
435. Crohn, Burrill, M.D. and Harry Yarnis, M.D. Regional Ileitis. 2nd Revised Edition, New York: Grune and Stratton, 1958 p. 121-123
436. British Medical Journal 2:762-764, 1979
437. Zeitschrift fur Gastroenterologie 19(1)6, January, 1981
438. American Journal of Clinical Nutrition 24:1068-1073, 1971
439. British Medical Journal 2:764-766, Sept. 29, 1979
440. Beeson. op. cit. p. 1560-1567
441. American Journal of Digestive Diseases 12:81, 1967
442. Howard, Rosanne, and Nancie Herbold. Nutrition in Clinical Care. New York: McGraw-Hill, 1978, p. 370
443. Modern Medicine, June, 1981, p. 42
444. Luckmann. op cit. p. 981-985
445. Hospital Medicine, February, 1979, p. 8-19
446. Journal of Urology 72:1057-1060, December, 1954
447. New England Journal of Medicine 298:856, April 13, 1978
448. Medical World News, July 20, 1962, p. 118
449. The Journal of Urology 125(1):51-54, January, 1981
450. British Journal of Urology 50:459-464, 1978
451. Family Practice News, May 15, 1981, p. 1,54
452. British Journal of Urology 51:427-431, 1979
453. British Journal of Urology 53(5)416-420, October, 1981
454. Brunner. op. cit. p. 509-510
455. British Medical Journal 1:802, June 24, 1967
456. The Lancet 2:401, August 19, 1967
457. Journal of the American Medical Association 226(8)1021, November 19, 1973
458. British Medical Journal 281:426, August 9, 1980
459. Luckmann. op. cit. p. 1271
460. British Medical Journal 2:1428-1491, December 12, 1964
461. The Lancet 2:1031-1034, November 2, 1974

462. British Medical Journal 2:149-152, July 16, 1977
463. Journal of Asthma Research 5(1)11-20, September, 1967
464. Journal of the American Medical Association 198(69)605-607, November 7, 1966
465. British Medical Journal 280:519-521, February 23, 1980
466. Family Practice News, April 15, 1979
467. Buchman. op. cit. p. 76, 77
468. Cumming, Gordon. Disorders of the Respiratory System. Oxford: Blackwell Scientific Pubs. 1973, p. 265
469. The Lancet 278:91, January 9, 1960
470. Phipps. op. cit.
471. Arthritis/Rheumatism Newsletter, August, 1979
472. Arthritis Newscard, November, 1980
473. Breneman, J. C. M.D. Basics of Food Allergy. Springfield: C. C. Thomas, 1978 pp. 84-91
474. Pediatrics 56:621, 1975
475. American Journal of Nursing 75(6)986-987, June, 1975
476. Scandinavian Journal of Rheumatology 1:61-64, 1972
477. Clinics in Experimental Immunology 9:677-693, 1971
478. Wyngaarden. op. cit. pp. 1800-1802
479. Annals of Allergy 39(1):8-11, July, 1977
480. Journal of the Minnesota Medical Association and the Northwestern Lancet, May 1, 1906
481. Graedon. op. cit. p. 164
482. Science News, August 12, 1939, p. 107
483. Journal of Family Practice 11(7)1041-1045, 1980
484. Postgraduate Medicine 67:117-130, June, 1980
485. Brunner. op. cit. p. 576-577
486. Pediatric Clinics of North America 20(4) 852-856, November, 1973
487. Journal of the American Medical Association 82(10)788-789, March 8, 1924
488. Journal of the American Medical Association 166(15)1862-1867, April 12, 1958
489. Luckmann. op. cit. pp. 1887-1890
490. Ginekologia Polska 46(4)405-408, April, 1975
491. Cutis 20:97-98, July, 1977
492. Physician Assistant and Health Practitioner September, 1980, p. 28-30
493. Physician and Sportsmedicine 9(6)43-54, June, 1981
494. The Medical Letter on Drugs and Therapeutics 19(8)33-34, April 22, 1977

495. Medical Tribune, January 12, 1977
496. American Family Physician, July, 1977 pp. 95-101
497. New England Journal of Medicine 294:172, January 15, 1976
498. Wyngaarden. op. cit. p. 2273
499. International Journal of Dermatology 17(5)380-387, June, 1978
500. Vaughn, Victor C., M.D., Et Al. Nelson Textbook of Pediatrics, 1979, pp. 1881-1882
501. Archives of Dermatology 112:1304-1307, September, 1976
502. American Journal of Nursing 71(11)2139-2140, November, 1971
503. The Lancet 1 (8273)663, March 20, 1982
504. Menkes, John H. Textbook of Child Neurology, 2nd Edition. Philadelphia: Lea and Febiger. 1980 p. 400-401
505. Actas Oto-Laryngologica 92:115-121, July-August, 1981
506. Brunner. op. cit. p. 205-210
507. Wyngaarden. op. cit. pp. 386-387
508. Luckmann. op. cit. p. 1269-1271
509. New England Journal of Medicine 247(15)557-567, October 9, 1952
510. American Journal of Epidemiology 90:390-399, November, 1969
511. Medical Journal of South Africa 14(8):398 March, 1919
512. Brunner. op. cit. 341-344
513. Luckmann. op. cit. pp. 1127-1132
514. American Journal of Clinical Nutrition 30:1963, 1977
515. New England Journal of Medicine 302:987-991 1980
516. American Journal of Diseases of Children 41:48-52, 1931
517. Journal of the American Medical Association 183(3):194-198, 1963
518. Angiology 2:138-140, 1951
519. British Journal of Surgery 60:187-190, March, 1973
520. Wyngaarden. op. cit. p. 328-331
521. Graedon. op. cit. p. 138-139
522. Archives of Physical Medicine and Rehabilitation 62:96, February, 1981
523. Buchman. op. cit. p. 102
524. Ibid. p. 124
525. Bricklin, Mark, Rodale's Encyclopedia of Natural Home Remedies. Emmaus, PA: Rodale Press, 1982 p. 83
526. The Lancet 2:379, August 22, 1981
527. The Lancet 2:381, August 22, 1981
528. Gastroenterology 82:638, April, 1982
529. Pediatrics 56(3)398-403, Sept. 1975

530. Chest 75:544-548, May, 1979
531. Journal of the American Geriatrics Society 11:570-573, 1963
532. Nutrition Today 6(6)8, November-December, 1971
533. Annals of Allergy 47:338-344, November, 1981
534. Journal of Laboratory and Clinical Medicine 22:921-924, June, 1934
535. Nutrition Today 11(1):6, January-February, 1976

INDEX FOR NATURAL REMEDIES

Abdominal breathing   17
Acetylsalicylic acid   14
Acid-ash   89
Acne, cystic   1
Acne vulgaris   1, 128
Acrodermatitis enteropathica   2
Alcoholic beverages   6, 7, 14, 60, 74, 82, 104, 121, 160
Alfalfa tea   48
Alkaline-ash   89
Alka-Seltzer   99
Allergic Rhinitis   62, 117
Almonds   101
Aloe vera   100, 115, 133
Aluminum   99
Alzheimer's Disease   99
Analgesics   76
Angina   3
Angina, nocturnal   5
Angina pectoris   3
Animal fat   47
Animal protein   54, 59, 74, 89
Anise tea   17, 30, 39, 57
Antacids   92, 97, 98, 99
Antibiotics   6, 45, 67, 83, 120, 122, 124, 133
Anti-gizzard erosion factor   99
Antihistamines   15, 29, 30
Aphthous ulcers   5, 41
Arthritis   6
Arthritis, Rheumatoid   110
Asparagus   79, 109
Aspirin   2, 15, 67, 76, 99
Asthma   10
Asthma, extrinsic   10
Asthma, intrinsic   10
Atherosclerosis   3
Athlete's foot   17
Avocados   82, 109

Backache   19, 70
Backache, foot exercise for   20

Bad breath   22, 70
Baking powder   47
Baking soda   47
Banana   15, 36, 37, 47, 56, 82, 103, 122, 133
Bands, tight   46, 55
Bedwetting   25
Beer   104
Bell's palsy   26
Bell's phenomenon   26
Berry, Dr. Maxwell   101
Birth control pills   45, 108
Bland diet   97, 98
Blood sugar levels   80, 101
Borgman, Dr. Robert   53
Boric acid   18
Bradykinesia   92
Bran   53, 73, 75
Bread, white   101
Breast cancer   91
Breast-feeding   2, 16, 36, 38, 76, 121
Breathing, abdominal or diaphragmatic   17, 29, 49, 95
Breathing exercises   68, 95, 114, 129
Bronchiectasis   28
Bronchitis   29
Buchu tea   45, 75, 79
Buerger's disease   31
Buerger's exercises   32, 86
Burdock tea   79
Burkitt, Dr. Denis   127
Bursitis   33
Butter fats   24

Cabbage   99, 109, 122, 133
Caffeine   82, 99, 109, 121
Calamine lotion   102
Calcium   2, 88, 89, 97
Calcium carbonate   98
Calcium oxalate   74
Candida albicans   119, 124
Canker sores   5
Carbohydrate refined   47, 53, 82

Carob 122
Carrots 122
Cataracts 11, 122
Catnip tea 12, 39, 51, 64, 123
Celery 100
Celiac disease 34
Cereals 14
Chamomile tea 15, 39, 45, 48, 51
Charcoal 24, 40, 43, 55, 59, 118, 122
Charcoal poultices 8, 27, 37, 59, 66
Cheese 8, 14, 72, 82, 121
Cherries 61
Chenodiol 54
Chenodeoxycholic acid 54
Chewing gum 6, 16, 56
Chiggers 36
Childers, Dr. Norman 6
Chilling 4, 15, 22, 26, 28, 29, 31, 32, 34, 44, 62, 67, 83, 85, 92,
    106, 116, 122
Chocolate 6, 7, 14, 25, 38, 47, 48, 50, 62, 71, 72, 75, 81, 82, 104,
    121
Cholecystectomy 54
Cholecystitis 51
Cholelithiasis 51
Cigarettes 92
Circadian rhythm 84, 98, 123
Citrus fruits 6, 25, 38, 62, 82, 104, 121
Clofibrate 52
Cockroaches 15
Coffee 7, 36, 38, 48, 71, 75, 82, 92, 99, 104, 109, 111, 121
Cola drinks 104, 121
Colchicine 60
Colic 37
Collateral circulation 32
Colon cancer 54
Colonic pressure 46
Comfrey 61, 78, 132
Constipation 25, 46, 47, 48, 49, 70, 73, 95, 100
Corn 7, 25, 36, 38, 44, 47, 53, 56, 62, 79, 82
Corn oil 90
Cornsilk tea 79
Cornstarch 18

Corticosteriods   11, 27, 43, 92, 122
Cortisone   7, 118, 212
Cosmetics   1
Cough suppressants   29, 30
Cradle cap   40
Cranberry juice   45
Crohn's disease   41
Cystitis   43

Decongestants   30
Dehydration   23, 96
Diabetes   11, 70, 109
Diplostreptococcus agalactiae   112
Diuretic teas   79
Diuretics   60
Diverticulitis   46
Diverticulosis   46
Diverticulum   46
Dopamine   93
Drafts   28
Drugs in labor and delivery   39
Duodenal ulcer   97, 99, 100
Dysmenorrhea   47

Eating between meals   99
Eczema   42
Egg   7, 14, 16, 25, 38, 40, 44, 50, 53, 62, 72, 79, 82, 111, 121
Elastic stockings   110, 128
Enuresis   24
Ergot   108
Egotamine tartrate   60
Estrogens   91
Ethacrynic acid   60
Eucalyptus   12, 30, 105
Exercise   3, 4, 12, 19, 22, 24, 25, 32, 47, 48, 52, 55, 62, 68, 72, 75, 80,
     83, 87, 91, 93, 94, 95, 101, 106, 110, 112, 113, 117, 118, 122, 123,
     127, 128
Expectorants   30

Fasting   58, 111, 131
Fats   5, 16, 32, 41, 53, 69, 70, 74, 82, 85, 90, 108, 132
Feingold, Dr. Ben   25
Ferrous sulphate   111

Fiber   42, 46, 47, 52, 73, 123, 127
Fish   38, 50, 53
Flagyl   125
Flat feet and backache   21
Flatulence   54
Fluoride   91, 99
Folic acid   60
Food allergies   6, 25
Food sensitivities   2
Foot exercise for low back pain   20

Gallstones   51
Garlic   12, 18, 36, 39, 46, 57, 82, 118, 120, 133
Gas   35, 39, 54, 70, 71, 100
Gas, cooking with   30
Gastric acid   97
Gastric ulcer   97, 99
Gastrin   97, 99
Girdles   17, 33, 46, 55, 125, 127, 131, 185
Gliaden   35
Gluten   35, 36, 42, 111, 121
Gold shots   7
Goldenseal   2, 6, 18, 45, 103, 105, 123
Gout   58
Grains   25, 36, 57, 74
Griseofulvin   18

Hair spray   17
Halitosis   22
Hammock   20
Hay fever   17, 25, 42, 62
Heat, moist   22, 31, 71, 114
Heating compress   31
Hemorrhoids   127
Heparin   92
Hiatus hernia   127
Hiccups   63
Homan's sign   130
Horseradish   42
Hydrochloric acid   100, 101
Hypertension   69
Hypoglycemic syndrome   101

Ice massage   22
Ice pack   22, 34, 114
Immunizations   8
Impetigo   65
Indian Dance   26
Indole   8
Influenza   66
Insulin   60
Intermittent claudication   31, 68
Irritable bowel syndrome   70
Itching   37
Itching, anal   103

Jewelweed   102

Kidney stones   59, 73
Knee-chest position   58

Lactose intolerance   43, 71, 104
Laxatives   55, 72, 104
L-dihydroxyphenylalanine   93
L-dopa   93
Lemon   102
Let's Have Healthy Children   39
Lettuce   100, 109
Levodopa   93

Margarine, polyunsaturated   90
Mastitis   76
Meals, heavy   4
Meat   89
Melons   15
Meniere's disease   78
Menthol   12
Methylxanthines   48
Migraine   53, 80
Milk   2, 7, 14, 16, 25, 30, 35, 36, 38, 40, 43, 50, 56, 61, 62, 71, 72, 74,
     79, 81, 87, 90, 97, 104, 111, 112, 121
Milk-alkali syndrome   74
Milk fats   24
Millet   101, 121
Mineral oil   104
Mint   45

Monosodium glutamate   51, 83
Morning sickness   49
Morning stiffness   7, 111, 114
Motion sickness remedies   109
Mouth breathing   14, 23
Mouth washes   6, 23, 29
Mud packs   60
Mullein tea   12
Muscle cramps   84
Muscle spasm   22, 95
Muscle strain   21
Mustard   42
Myocardial infarction   91, 97

Nasal congestion   62, 67, 116
Nebulizers   12
Neutral bath   12
Nicotine   108
Nightshades   7, 111
Norephinephrine   82

Oatmeal   103
Olives   101
Onions   32, 38, 56, 82
Oral Contraceptives   52, 81, 124, 127, 130
Orange   82
Osteoarthritis   6
Osteoporosis   87, 122
Overeating   43, 50, 57, 61, 72, 121

Paraffin bath   115
Parathyroid hormone   91
Parkinson's disease   92
Parsley tea   45
Passive smokers   108
Pecans   7
Pepper   42
Peppermint   39, 51, 86, 117, 123
Peptic ulcer   97, 122
Perfume   17
Periodontal disease   89
Phlebothrombosis   130

Phosphorus   89, 99
Plantain   102
Plums   82
Poison ivy   101
Pork   7, 53, 72, 82
Postural drainage   13
Posture   50, 94, 114
Potato   101, 109, 133
Prednisone   28
Prostaglandins   99
Protein   89
Protein, high   8, 130
Prurines   59, 74
Pruritus ani   103

Raspberries   82
Raynaud's disease   105
Raynaud's phenomenon   31, 105
Red raspberry leaf tea   48
Regional enteritis   41
Renal calculi   73
Restless leg syndrome   109
Rheumatoid arthritis   6, 110
Ringworm of the feet   17

Sage   129
Saline   6, 18, 102, 116, 125
Salt   2, 50, 79, 83, 85, 102, 110, 112, 116, 131
"Silent" gallstones   52
Simethicone   57
Sinusitis   23, 115
Sippy diet   97
Sitz bath   45, 50, 104, 122, 125
Skatole   8
Sleep breathing   15
Slippery elm bark   123
Slurry water   122
Smoking   4, 6, 16, 21, 28, 30, 32, 51, 56, 68, 72, 79, 82, 83, 91, 99, 108, 116
Soda pop   89
Soda water   125
Sodium   98
Sodium benzoate   11, 14

Sodium bicarbonate 99
Sodium fluoride 91
Sodium glutamate 83
Sodium metabisulfite 11, 14
Sodium nitrite 83
Soft drinks 109
Sorbitol 57
Sore throat 67
Soy milk protein 2
Soy protein intolerance 35
Soy sauce 51
Spastic colon 70
Spearmint tea 57
Spermaticides 45
Spices 47, 53, 104
Steroids 99, 120, 124
Stomach acid 98
Stress 1, 32, 42, 57, 69, 72, 83, 106, 109, 122
Stroke 91
Sucrose 89
Sugar 1, 42, 44, 47, 66, 68, 69, 73, 85, 100, 108, 111
Support hose 128
Sulfa 60
Sulfur-dioxide 14
Sunlight 65, 91, 109, 124, 125, 134
Svartz, Nanna 112
Synthetic fabrics 14, 18, 105, 125

Tallow 90
Tartrazine 11, 14, 83
Tea 7, 48, 71, 75, 77, 82, 109, 121
Tennis elbow 118
Terezakis, Nia K. M.D. 1
Tetracycline 125, 133
Thiamine chloride 60
Thiazides 60
Thromboangiitis obliterans 31
Thrombophlebitis—See Venous thrombosis 130
Thrush 119
Thyme 17, 24, 39, 57
Tinea pedis 17
Tinnitis 78, 80
Tobacco 7

Tomato   7, 104, 121
Toothpaste   6, 23
Tophi   58
Trichomonas vaginalis   124
Triglycerides   108
Tyramine   82
Tyrosine   82

Ulcerative colitis   41, 120
Ulcers   97
Urate   58
Uric acid   58, 60, 74
Urogastrone   99
Urolithiasis   59, 73
Urushiol   101
Uvula   64

Vaccines   6, 15
Vaginitis   124
Vaporizer   28, 30
Varicose veins   87, 126
Vaseline milk   96
Vegan diet   5
Venous stasis   110
Venous thrombosis   130
Vertigo   78, 80
Vinegar   14, 18, 42, 47, 83, 103
Vinegar douche   125
Vitamin B   52, 82
Vitamin B-6   93
Vitamin B-12   60
Vitamin C   52, 75, 91, 101
Vitamin D   74, 90
Vitamin E   109
Vitamin U   99

Warts   132
Watermelon seed tea   79
Wheat   7, 35, 40, 50, 57, 72, 79, 82, 111, 121
Whedon, G. Donald   88
Worcestershire sauce   51, 75

Xylitol   57

Yeast   45, 60, 79, 82, 119

Zinc absorption   2
Zinc deficiency   3

ORDER FORM

Of These Ye May Freely Eat Cookbook- J. Rachor	2.95
Of These Ye May Freely Eat Supplement on Practical Instructions in Cooking & Nutrition- J. Rachor	2.95
Natural Remedies- Agatha & Calvin Thrash, M.D.	6.95
More Natural Remedies- Agatha & Calvin Thrash, M.D.	6.95
Nutrition For Vegetarians- Agatha & Calvin Thrash,MD	9.95
Home Remedies- Agatha & Calvin Thrash, M.D.	9.95
Rx Charcoal- Agatha & Calvin Thrash, M.D.	6.95
Food Alleregies Made Simple- Thrash, M.D.	4.95
Animal Connection- Agatha & Calvin Thrash, M.D.	4.95
Premenstrual Syndrome (PMS)- Thrash, M.D.	2.95
Problems With Meat- John Scharffenberg, M.D.	4.95
Sunlight- Zane Kime, M.D.	12.95
New Start- Vernon Foster- M.D.	9.95
To Your Health- Dr. Hans Diehl	9.95
Home Made Health- Raymond & Dorthy Moore	9.95
Diet, Crime & Delinquency- Alexander Schauss	5.95
How To Stop Smoking- Magazine	2.50
Eat For Strength Cookbook- Agatha Thrash, M.D.	7.95
Eat For Strength Cookbook (no oil)- Thrash, M.D.	7.95
Joy of Cooking Naturally Cookbook- Peggy Dameron	9.95
Cooking With Natural Foods- M. Beltz, Black Hills	14.95
Recipes from the Weimar Kitchen- Weimar Inst.	9.95
The Eight Doctors music tape- Jennifer Schwizer	4.95

NAME _____   Subtotal   _____

ADDRESS_____   Postage ($1.25 1st
                                 item, .35 ea. add.)

                                             _____

_____   Tax (4% Mich _____
                                     res.)
Mail To: Family Health Publ.
          13062 Musgrove Hwy.
          Sunfield, MI   48890 Total   _____